Welcome to **The Complete Cookbook for Young Chefs**, your ultimate guide to mastering the art of cooking with ease, creativity, and confidence! Whether you are just starting your culinary journey or looking to expand your kitchen skills, this cookbook is designed with you in mind. Packed with over 115 mouthwatering recipes, this book is your ticket to creating delicious, nutritious meals that will impress your family and friends.

Cooking should be fun and accessible, which is why we've crafted recipes that are not only simple to follow but also bursting with flavor and nutritional value. From breakfast delights to satisfying dinners and delectable desserts, you'll find a diverse range of dishes that cater to various tastes and dietary preferences.

Each recipe comes with step-by-step instructions, helpful tips, and vibrant photos to guide you through the cooking process. We've also included essential cooking techniques, safety tips, and advice on selecting the best ingredients, ensuring you build a solid foundation in the kitchen.

This cookbook isn't just about making meals; it's about discovering the joy of cooking, experimenting with new flavors, and developing skills that will last a lifetime. So grab your apron, gather your ingredients, and get ready to conquer the kitchen with confidence. Your culinary adventure starts here!

Happy cooking!

1. Avocado Toast with Poached Egg

Ingredient:

• 2 slices of whole grain or sourdough bread
• 1 ripe avocado, mashed
• 2 eggs
• 1 tbsp white vinegar
• Salt and pepper to taste
• Optional toppings: cherry tomatoes, microgreens, red pepper flakes

Instructions:

1. Fill a medium saucepan with 3•4 inches of water and bring to a gentle simmer over medium heat. Add the white vinegar.

2. Crack the eggs one at a time into a small bowl or ramekin. Gently slide the eggs from the bowl into the simmering water. Poach the eggs for 3•5 minutes, until the whites are set but the yolks are still runny.

3. While the eggs are poaching, toast the bread slices until golden brown.

4. Spread the mashed avocado evenly over the toasted bread slices.

5. Using a slotted spoon, carefully remove the poached eggs from the water and place one on top of each avocado toast.

6. Season with salt and pepper to taste.

7. Top with any additional desired toppings like cherry tomatoes, microgreens, or red pepper flakes.

Serve the avocado toast with poached egg immediately while the egg is still warm. This is a nutritious and delicious breakfast or snack that young chefs can easily assemble.

2. Banana Oat Pancakes

Ingredient:

- 1 cup rolled oats
- 1 ripe banana, mashed
- 2 eggs
- 1/4 cup milk of your choice
- 1 tsp baking powder
- 1/4 tsp cinnamon (optional)
- Pinch of salt
- Butter or oil for cooking

Toppings (optional):
- Maple syrup
- Fresh fruit (berries, sliced banana, etc.)
- Nut butter
- Whipped cream

Instructions:

1. In a medium bowl, mash the ripe banana until smooth.

2. Add the rolled oats, eggs, milk, baking powder, cinnamon (if using), and a pinch of salt. Stir until well combined.

3. Heat a skillet or griddle over medium heat and grease with a small amount of butter or oil.

4. Scoop about 1/4 cup of the batter onto the hot surface, forming pancakes. Cook for 2•3 minutes per side, or until golden brown.

5. Flip the pancakes carefully using a spatula. Cook the other side for an additional 2•3 minutes.

6. Serve the banana oat pancakes warm, with your desired toppings. Maple syrup, fresh fruit, nut butter, and whipped cream are all delicious options.

These pancakes are a great way to get kids involved in the kitchen. They're easy to make, nutritious, and fun to customize with different toppings.

3. Spinach and Feta Omelette

Ingredient:

- 2 eggs
- 1 tbsp milk or water
- 1 cup fresh spinach, washed and chopped
- 2 tbsp crumbled feta cheese
- 1 tsp butter or oil for cooking
- Salt and pepper to taste

Instructions:

1. Crack the eggs into a small bowl and beat them lightly with a fork or whisk. Add the milk or water and a pinch of salt and pepper, then whisk to combine.

2. Heat a small non•stick skillet over medium heat and melt the butter or heat the oil.

3. Pour the egg mixture into the hot pan and let it sit for 20•30 seconds to set the bottom.

4. Using a spatula, gently push the cooked egg from the edges into the center, tilting the pan to allow the uncooked egg to flow to the edges. Do this all the way around the pan.

5. When the eggs are mostly set but still a bit runny on top, sprinkle the chopped spinach and crumbled feta cheese over half of the omelette.

6. Use the spatula to fold the unfilled half of the omelette over the filled half.

7. Slide the omelette onto a plate and serve immediately.

Tips for young chefs:
- Be careful when cracking the eggs to avoid getting any shell in the bowl.
- Use a non•stick pan to make the omelette easy to flip.
- Take your time when folding the omelette to keep it intact.

Enjoy your delicious spinach and feta omelette!

4. Greek Yogurt with Honey and Berries

Ingredient:

• 1 cup plain Greek yogurt
• 2 tbsp honey
• 1 cup mixed berries (such as blueberries, raspberries, and/or strawberries)

Instructions:

1. Scoop the Greek yogurt into a bowl or serving dish.

2. Drizzle the honey over the top of the yogurt.

3. Gently fold the honey into the yogurt using a spoon, creating a swirled effect.

4. Top the honey•yogurt mixture with the mixed berries.

That's it! This healthy and delicious snack or breakfast is ready to enjoy.

Tips for young chefs:

• Let the young chef measure out the yogurt, honey, and berries. This helps them practice their measuring skills.

• Encourage them to gently fold the honey into the yogurt to create a nice swirled pattern.

• Suggest they try different types of berries or even other fresh fruit like sliced bananas or kiwi.

• Talk about the different flavors and textures they experience as they eat the yogurt, honey, and berries.

This recipe is simple, nutritious, and a great way to get kids involved in the kitchen. Enjoy!

5. Breakfast Burrito

Ingredient:

- 2 eggs, scrambled
- 2 tbsp shredded cheddar cheese
- 2 tbsp diced bell pepper (any color)
- 2 tbsp diced onion
- 1 small flour tortilla
- Salt and pepper to taste
- Optional toppings: salsa, avocado, sour cream

Instructions:

1. In a small non•stick skillet, scramble the eggs over medium heat until cooked through. Season with a pinch of salt and pepper.

2. Remove the scrambled eggs from the pan and place them in a bowl.

3. In the same skillet, sauté the diced bell pepper and onion over medium heat for 2•3 minutes, until softened.

4. Add the sautéed veggies to the bowl with the scrambled eggs. Sprinkle the shredded cheddar cheese on top and gently mix everything together.

5. Warm the flour tortilla according to package instructions, either in the microwave for 20•30 seconds or in a dry skillet for 30 seconds per side.

6. Spoon the egg, veggie, and cheese mixture onto the center of the warm tortilla.

7. Fold the bottom of the tortilla up, then fold in the sides and continue rolling it up into a burrito shape.

8. Serve the breakfast burrito warm, with any desired toppings like salsa, avocado, or sour cream.

Tips for young chefs:
- Let them help scramble the eggs and sauté the veggies.
- Encourage them to customize the fillings with their favorite ingredients.
- Show them how to properly fold and roll the burrito.

This breakfast burrito is a tasty and portable meal that kids will love!

6. Smoothie Bowl with Granola

Ingredient:

• 1 cup frozen mixed berries (such as strawberries, blueberries, and raspberries)
• 1 banana, frozen
• 1/2 cup milk of your choice (dairy, almond, oat, etc.)
• 1/4 cup plain Greek yogurt
• 1 tbsp honey (optional)
• 1/4 cup granola
• Fresh fruit for topping (sliced banana, berries, etc.)

Instructions:

1. In a blender, combine the frozen mixed berries, frozen banana, milk, and Greek yogurt. Blend until smooth and creamy.

2. If desired, add the honey and blend again briefly to incorporate.

3. Pour the smoothie into a bowl.

4. Sprinkle the granola evenly over the top of the smoothie.

5. Arrange the fresh fruit toppings, such as sliced banana and berries, around the edges of the bowl.

Tips for young chefs:
• Let them measure and add the ingredients to the blender.
• Encourage them to blend the smoothie until it's nice and smooth.
• Have them carefully pour the smoothie into the bowl.
• Allow them to sprinkle the granola and arrange the fresh fruit toppings.

This Smoothie Bowl with Granola is a nutritious and delicious breakfast or snack that's fun for kids to make. The creamy smoothie, crunchy granola, and fresh fruit create a tasty and visually appealing dish. Enjoy!

7. French Toast

Ingredient:

- 3 eggs
- 1/2 cup milk
- 1 tsp vanilla extract
- 1/2 tsp ground cinnamon
- Pinch of salt
- 6 slices of bread (such as challah, brioche, or sourdough)
- Butter or oil for cooking
- Maple syrup, powdered sugar, or other toppings (optional)

Instructions:

1. In a shallow bowl, whisk together the eggs, milk, vanilla, cinnamon, and salt until well combined.

2. Dip each slice of bread into the egg mixture, coating both sides evenly.

3. Heat a large skillet or griddle over medium heat and melt a small amount of butter or heat a drizzle of oil.

4. Working in batches, place the soaked bread slices onto the hot surface and cook for 2•3 minutes per side, or until golden brown.

5. Flip the slices carefully using a spatula.

6. Once both sides are cooked, transfer the French toast to a plate.

7. Serve the French toast warm, with your desired toppings such as maple syrup, powdered sugar, fresh fruit, or whipped cream.

Tips for young chefs:
- Let them help measure and whisk the egg mixture.
- Encourage them to dip the bread slices into the egg mixture.
- Have them carefully place the soaked bread onto the hot surface.
- Let them sprinkle on the toppings of their choice.

French toast is a classic breakfast that kids love to make and eat. The combination of the sweet, custard•like interior and the crispy exterior is simply delicious. Enjoy!

8. Chia Seed Pudding

Ingredient:

• 1/4 cup chia seeds
• 1 cup milk of your choice (dairy, almond, oat, etc.)
• 2 tbsp honey or maple syrup (optional)
• 1/2 tsp vanilla extract (optional)
• Pinch of cinnamon (optional)
• Fresh fruit for topping (berries, sliced banana, etc.)

Instructions:

1. In a medium bowl or mason jar, combine the chia seeds and milk. Stir well to combine.

2. If using, add the honey or maple syrup and vanilla extract. Stir again until everything is well mixed.

3. Cover the bowl or seal the mason jar and refrigerate for at least 2 hours, or overnight. The chia seeds will thicken the mixture into a pudding•like consistency.

4. When ready to serve, give the chia pudding a good stir to incorporate any liquid that has separated.

5. Spoon the chia pudding into bowls or cups. Top with your desired fresh fruit.

6. If you'd like, sprinkle a pinch of cinnamon over the top.

Tips for young chefs:
• Let them measure and add the chia seeds and milk.
• Encourage them to experiment with different types of milk and sweeteners.
• Have them help stir the mixture before refrigerating.
• Let them choose and arrange the fresh fruit toppings.

Chia seed pudding is a nutritious and delicious breakfast or snack that's easy for kids to make. The chia seeds provide fiber, protein, and omega•3s, while the fruit adds natural sweetness and vitamins. Enjoy!

9. Veggie Breakfast Hash

Ingredient:

• 2 medium potatoes, diced
• 1 bell pepper, diced
• 1 onion, diced
• 2 cloves garlic, minced
• 1 cup diced mushrooms
• 2 eggs
• 2 tbsp olive oil
• Salt and pepper to taste
• Optional toppings: shredded cheese, chopped fresh herbs, hot sauce

Instructions:

1. In a large skillet, heat the olive oil over medium heat.

2. Add the diced potatoes, bell pepper, onion, and garlic to the skillet. Cook for 8•10 minutes, stirring occasionally, until the vegetables are starting to soften.

3. Stir in the diced mushrooms and continue cooking for another 5•7 minutes, until the potatoes are tender and the vegetables are lightly browned.

4. Create two small wells in the hash and crack the eggs directly into them. Cover the skillet and cook for 3•5 minutes, or until the egg whites are set but the yolks are still runny.

5. Remove the skillet from the heat and season the hash with salt and pepper to taste.

6. Serve the Veggie Breakfast Hash warm, with the eggs on top. Add any desired toppings like shredded cheese, chopped fresh herbs, or hot sauce.

Tips for young chefs:
• Let them help dice the potatoes, bell pepper, onion, and mushrooms.
• Encourage them to carefully crack the eggs into the wells in the hash.
• Have them sprinkle on the salt and pepper, and any other toppings.

This Veggie Breakfast Hash is a nutritious and flavorful meal that's perfect for breakfast or brunch. The combination of roasted vegetables and runny eggs makes it a delicious and satisfying dish for young chefs to prepare.

10. Blueberry Muffins

Ingredient:
- 1 1/2 cups all•purpose flour
- 3/4 cup granulated sugar
- 1 1/2 tsp baking powder
- 1/4 tsp salt
- 1/2 cup milk
- 1/3 cup vegetable oil
- 1 egg
- 1 tsp vanilla extract
- 1 cup fresh or frozen blueberries

Instructions:

1. Preheat your oven to 400°F (200°C). Grease a 12•cup muffin tin or line it with paper liners.

2. In a large bowl, whisk together the flour, sugar, baking powder, and salt.

3. In a separate bowl, whisk together the milk, vegetable oil, egg, and vanilla extract.

4. Gently fold the wet ingredients into the dry ingredients, being careful not to overmix. Fold in the blueberries.

5. Scoop the batter evenly into the prepared muffin cups, filling them about 3/4 full.

6. Bake for 18•20 minutes, or until a toothpick inserted into the center comes out clean.

7. Allow the muffins to cool in the tin for 5 minutes, then transfer them to a wire rack to cool completely.

Tips for young chefs:
- Let them help measure and mix the dry ingredients.
- Encourage them to gently fold in the wet ingredients and blueberries.
- Have them use an ice cream scoop or large spoon to portion the batter into the muffin cups.
- Assist them in checking the muffins for doneness and transferring them to the cooling rack.

These Blueberry Muffins are a delicious and easy•to•make treat that kids will love. The sweet, juicy blueberries and tender muffin texture make them a perfect breakfast or snack. Enjoy!

11. Overnight Oats

Ingredient:

- 1/2 cup rolled oats
- 1/2 cup milk of your choice (dairy, almond, oat, etc.)
- 2 tbsp plain Greek yogurt
- 1 tbsp chia seeds (optional)
- 1 tbsp honey or maple syrup (optional)
- 1/4 tsp vanilla extract (optional)
- Pinch of cinnamon (optional)
- Fresh fruit for topping (berries, sliced banana, etc.)

Instructions:

1. In a mason jar or small bowl, combine the rolled oats, milk, Greek yogurt, chia seeds (if using), honey or maple syrup (if using), and vanilla extract (if using).

2. Stir all the ingredients together until well combined.

3. Cover the jar or bowl and refrigerate overnight, or for at least 4 hours.

4. In the morning, give the overnight oats a good stir. The oats will have absorbed the liquid and become thick and creamy.

5. Top the overnight oats with your desired fresh fruit, a sprinkle of cinnamon, or any other toppings you like.

Tips for young chefs:
- Let them measure and add the oats, milk, and other ingredients.
- Encourage them to experiment with different types of milk, yogurt, and sweeteners.
- Have them help stir the mixture before refrigerating.
- Let them choose and arrange the fresh fruit toppings.

Overnight oats are a nutritious and delicious breakfast that's easy for kids to make. The oats provide fiber and complex carbs, while the yogurt and fruit add protein, vitamins, and natural sweetness. Enjoy!

12. Breakfast Quesadilla

Ingredient:

- 2 eggs, scrambled
- 2 tbsp shredded cheddar or Monterey Jack cheese
- 2 tbsp diced bell pepper
- 2 tbsp diced onion
- 1 small flour tortilla
- 1 tsp butter or oil for cooking

Optional Toppings:

- Salsa
- Sour cream
- Avocado

Instructions:

1. In a small non•stick skillet, scramble the eggs over medium heat until cooked through. Season with a pinch of salt and pepper.

2. Remove the scrambled eggs from the pan and place them in a bowl.

3. In the same skillet, sauté the diced bell pepper and onion over medium heat for 2•3 minutes, until softened.

4. Add the sautéed veggies to the bowl with the scrambled eggs. Sprinkle the shredded cheese on top and gently mix everything together.

5. Wipe the skillet clean and place it back over medium heat. Add the butter or oil.

6. Lay the flour tortilla in the hot skillet. Spoon the egg, veggie, and cheese mixture onto one half of the tortilla.

7. Fold the other half of the tortilla over the filled half to create a half•moon shape.

8. Cook the quesadilla for 2•3 minutes per side, or until the tortilla is golden brown and the cheese is melted.

9. Remove the quesadilla from the skillet and slice it in half. Serve the breakfast quesadilla warm, with any desired toppings like salsa, sour cream, or avocado.

Tips for young chefs:
- Let them help scramble the eggs and sauté the veggies.

13. Pumpkin Spice Waffles

Ingredient:

- 1 1/2 cups all•purpose flour
- 3 1/2 tsp baking powder
- 1 tsp ground cinnamon
- 1/2 tsp ground ginger
- 1/4 tsp ground nutmeg
- 1/4 tsp ground cloves
- 1/4 tsp salt
- 1 cup milk
- 1/2 cup pumpkin puree

- 2 tbsp brown sugar
- 2 tbsp vegetable oil
- 1 egg
- 1 tsp vanilla extract

Toppings (optional):
- Maple syrup
- Whipped cream
- Chopped pecans
- Powdered sugar

Instructions:

1. Preheat your waffle iron according to the manufacturer's instructions.

2. In a large bowl, whisk together the flour, baking powder, cinnamon, ginger, nutmeg, cloves, and salt.

3. In a separate bowl, whisk together the milk, pumpkin puree, brown sugar, vegetable oil, egg, and vanilla extract.

4. Gently fold the wet ingredients into the dry ingredients, being careful not to overmix.

5. Grease the preheated waffle iron and scoop the batter onto the hot surface, using about 1/2 cup of batter per waffle.

6. Cook the waffles for 3•5 minutes, or until they are golden brown and crispy.

7. Carefully remove the waffles from the iron and place them on a plate or wire rack.

8. Serve the pumpkin spice waffles warm, with your desired toppings such as maple syrup, whipped cream, chopped pecans, or powdered sugar.

Tips for young chefs:
- Let them help measure and mix the dry and wet ingredients.
- Encourage them to gently fold the wet ingredients into the dry ingredients.
- Have them use a ladle or measuring cup to scoop the batter onto the hot waffle iron.
- Allow them to choose and arrange the toppings.

14. Egg and Veggie Muffins

Ingredient:

- 6 eggs
- 1/2 cup diced bell pepper
- 1/2 cup diced onion
- 1/2 cup diced mushrooms
- 1/4 cup shredded cheddar cheese
- 2 tbsp milk
- Salt and pepper to taste
- Nonstick cooking spray

Instructions:

1. Preheat your oven to 350°F (175°C). Grease a 6•cup muffin tin with nonstick cooking spray.

2. In a medium bowl, whisk the eggs together with the milk. Season with a pinch of salt and pepper.

3. Stir in the diced bell pepper, onion, and mushrooms.

4. Divide the egg mixture evenly among the prepared muffin cups, filling them about 3/4 full.

5. Sprinkle the shredded cheddar cheese on top of each muffin.

6. Bake for 20•25 minutes, or until the eggs are set and the tops are lightly golden.

7. Remove the muffins from the oven and let them cool in the tin for 5 minutes.

8. Carefully transfer the egg muffins to a wire rack to cool completely.

Tips for young chefs:
- Let them help whisk the eggs and milk.
- Encourage them to stir in the diced vegetables.
- Have them use a spoon or ladle to portion the egg mixture into the muffin cups.
- Allow them to sprinkle the cheese on top of the muffins.

These Egg and Veggie Muffins are a nutritious and portable breakfast or snack that kids can easily make. The combination of eggs, veggies, and cheese makes them a tasty and satisfying option. Enjoy!

15. Peanut Butter Banana Smoothie

Ingredient:

- 1 ripe banana, frozen
- 1/2 cup milk of your choice (dairy, almond, oat, etc.)
- 2 tbsp peanut butter
- 1 tbsp honey (optional)
- 1/2 tsp vanilla extract
- Pinch of cinnamon (optional)
- Ice cubes (optional)

Instructions:

1. In a blender, combine the frozen banana, milk, peanut butter, honey (if using), vanilla extract, and cinnamon (if using).

2. Blend the ingredients on high speed until the mixture is smooth and creamy.

3. If you'd like a thicker consistency, add a few ice cubes and blend again briefly.

4. Pour the peanut butter banana smoothie into a glass.

5. Serve the smoothie immediately, with an optional garnish of a banana slice or a sprinkle of cinnamon.

Tips for young chefs:
- Let them measure and add the ingredients to the blender.
- Encourage them to blend the smoothie until it's nice and smooth.
- Have them pour the smoothie into a glass.
- Allow them to add any optional toppings or garnishes.

This Peanut Butter Banana Smoothie is a delicious and nutritious treat that's perfect for breakfast, a snack, or even dessert. The combination of creamy peanut butter, sweet banana, and milk creates a rich and satisfying smoothie that kids will love. Enjoy!

16. Chicken Caesar Salad

Ingredient:

• 2 boneless, skinless chicken breasts
• 1 tbsp olive oil
• Salt and pepper to taste
• 4 cups chopped romaine lettuce
• 1/4 cup shredded Parmesan cheese
• 1/4 cup Caesar salad dressing
• 1/2 cup croutons
• Lemon wedges for serving (optional)

Instructions:

1. Preheat your oven to 400°F (200°C).

2. Season the chicken breasts with salt and pepper on both sides.

3. Heat the olive oil in a large oven•safe skillet over medium•high heat. Add the chicken and cook for 3•4 minutes per side, until lightly browned.

4. Transfer the skillet to the preheated oven and bake the chicken for 12•15 minutes, or until it's cooked through and reaches an internal temperature of 165°F (75°C).

5. Remove the chicken from the oven and let it rest for 5 minutes. Then, slice or shred the chicken into bite•sized pieces.

6. In a large salad bowl, combine the chopped romaine lettuce, shredded Parmesan cheese, and croutons.

7. Drizzle the Caesar salad dressing over the salad and toss gently to coat.

8. Top the salad with the sliced or shredded chicken.

9. Serve the Chicken Caesar Salad immediately, with lemon wedges on the side if desired.

Tips for young chefs:
• Let them help measure and season the chicken.
• Encourage them to tear or chop the romaine lettuce.
• Have them sprinkle the Parmesan cheese and croutons over the salad.
• Assist them in drizzling the dressing and tossing the salad.

17. Quinoa and Black Bean Salad

Ingredient:

• 1 cup cooked quinoa, cooled
• 1 (15 oz) can black beans, rinsed and drained
• 1 cup diced cucumber
• 1/2 cup diced bell pepper
• 1/4 cup diced red onion
• 2 tbsp chopped fresh cilantro (or parsley)
• 2 tbsp lime juice
• 1 tbsp olive oil
• 1 tsp honey (optional)
• Salt and pepper to taste

Instructions:

1. In a large bowl, combine the cooked and cooled quinoa, black beans, diced cucumber, bell pepper, red onion, and chopped cilantro or parsley.

2. In a small bowl, whisk together the lime juice, olive oil, and honey (if using).

3. Pour the dressing over the quinoa and bean mixture and gently toss to coat everything evenly.

4. Season the salad with salt and pepper to taste.

5. Cover the bowl and refrigerate the quinoa and black bean salad for at least 30 minutes to allow the flavors to meld.

6. Serve the salad chilled or at room temperature.

Tips for young chefs:
• Let them help measure and add the quinoa, black beans, and chopped vegetables.
• Encourage them to whisk the dressing ingredients together.
• Have them gently toss the salad to combine the dressing.
• Allow them to season the salad with salt and pepper.

This Quinoa and Black Bean Salad is a nutritious and flavorful dish that's perfect for a light lunch or side. The combination of protein•rich quinoa, fiber•filled black beans, and fresh veggies makes it a great option for young chefs to prepare.

18. Turkey and Avocado Wrap

Ingredient:

• 1 whole wheat tortilla or wrap
• 2•3 slices of deli turkey
• 1/2 avocado, sliced
• 1•2 tbsp hummus
• 1/4 cup shredded lettuce or spinach
• 1 tbsp diced tomatoes (optional)
• Salt and pepper to taste

Instructions:

1. Lay the whole wheat tortilla or wrap on a clean surface.

2. Spread the hummus evenly over the center of the tortilla.

3. Layer the deli turkey slices on top of the hummus.

4. Arrange the avocado slices on top of the turkey.

5. Sprinkle the shredded lettuce or spinach over the avocado.

6. If using, add the diced tomatoes.

7. Season with a pinch of salt and pepper.

8. Fold the bottom of the tortilla up, then fold in the sides and continue rolling it up into a wrap shape.

9. Cut the wrap in half diagonally, if desired, and serve.

Tips for young chefs:
• Let them spread the hummus on the tortilla.
• Encourage them to layer the turkey, avocado, and greens.
• Have them sprinkle the tomatoes and season with salt and pepper.
• Show them how to properly fold and roll the wrap.

This Turkey and Avocado Wrap is a delicious and nutritious lunch or snack that's easy for kids to assemble. The combination of savory turkey, creamy avocado, and crunchy veggies makes it a tasty and satisfying option.

19. Vegetable Stir·Fry

Ingredient:

• 2 cups mixed vegetables (such as broccoli florets, sliced carrots, snow peas, and diced bell pepper)
• 1 tbsp vegetable oil
• 2 cloves garlic, minced
• 1 tsp grated ginger (optional)
• 2 tbsp soy sauce or tamari
• 1 tsp honey or brown sugar (optional)
• Salt and pepper to taste
• Cooked rice or noodles, for serving (optional)

Instructions:

1. Prepare all the vegetables by chopping or slicing them into bite·sized pieces.

2. In a large skillet or wok, heat the vegetable oil over medium·high heat.

3. Add the minced garlic and grated ginger (if using) to the hot oil. Stir·fry for 30 seconds to 1 minute, until fragrant.

4. Add the prepared vegetables to the skillet or wok. Stir·fry for 5·7 minutes, or until the vegetables are tender·crisp.

5. Pour in the soy sauce and honey or brown sugar (if using). Stir to coat the vegetables evenly.

6. Season with salt and pepper to taste.

7. Serve the vegetable stir·fry immediately, over cooked rice or noodles if desired.

Tips for young chefs:
• Let them help wash, chop, and slice the vegetables.
• Encourage them to measure and add the oil, garlic, and ginger.
• Have them pour in the soy sauce and sweetener, and stir to combine.
• Assist them in seasoning the stir·fry with salt and pepper.

This Vegetable Stir·Fry is a quick, healthy, and delicious meal that's perfect for young chefs to prepare. The combination of fresh vegetables, savory soy sauce, and a touch of sweetness makes it a family·friendly dish. Enjoy!

20. Tomato Basil Soup

Ingredient:

- 1 tbsp olive oil
- 1 onion, diced
- 3 cloves garlic, minced
- 1 (28 oz) can diced tomatoes
- 2 cups vegetable or chicken broth
- 1/4 cup fresh basil leaves, chopped
- 1 tsp sugar
- Salt and pepper to taste
- Croutons or grilled cheese sandwiches for serving (optional)

Instructions:

1. In a large pot or Dutch oven, heat the olive oil over medium heat.

2. Add the diced onion and sauté for 5•7 minutes, until softened and translucent.

3. Stir in the minced garlic and cook for an additional 1•2 minutes, until fragrant.

4. Pour in the can of diced tomatoes, including the juices, and the vegetable or chicken broth. Bring the mixture to a simmer.

5. Reduce the heat to low and let the soup simmer for 15•20 minutes, stirring occasionally.

6. Remove the pot from the heat and use an immersion blender to puree the soup until smooth. (Alternatively, you can carefully transfer the soup to a blender and blend in batches.)

7. Stir in the chopped fresh basil and sugar. Season with salt and pepper to taste.

8. Serve the tomato basil soup warm, with croutons or grilled cheese sandwiches on the side, if desired.

Tips for young chefs:
- Let them help measure and add the ingredients to the pot.
- Encourage them to stir the soup as it simmers.
- Have them use the immersion blender (with adult supervision) to puree the soup.
- Allow them to add the basil and season the soup with salt and pepper.

21. Grilled Cheese Sandwich

Ingredient:

• 2 slices of bread (white, whole wheat, or sourdough)
• 2•3 slices of cheddar, Swiss, or American cheese
• 1•2 tbsp butter or margarine

Instructions:

1. Heat a skillet or griddle over medium heat.

2. Butter one side of each slice of bread.

3. Place one slice of bread, butter•side down, in the hot skillet.

4. Layer the cheese slices on top of the bread.

5. Top with the other slice of bread, butter•side up.

6. Cook the sandwich for 2•3 minutes per side, or until the bread is golden brown and the cheese is melted.

7. Carefully flip the sandwich using a spatula and cook the other side.

8. Remove the grilled cheese sandwich from the skillet and let it cool for a minute before serving.

Tips for young chefs:
• Let them butter the bread slices.
• Encourage them to carefully layer the cheese slices.
• Have them place the sandwich in the hot skillet and monitor the cooking.
• Assist them in flipping the sandwich with a spatula.

This classic Grilled Cheese Sandwich is a simple and delicious meal that's perfect for young chefs to make. The combination of crispy, buttery bread and melted cheese is a crowd•pleaser. Serve it with a side of tomato soup for a comforting and satisfying lunch or dinner.

22. Chicken and Vegetable Skewers

Ingredient:

• 1 lb boneless, skinless chicken breasts, cut into 1•inch cubes
• 1 red bell pepper, cut into 1•inch pieces
• 1 zucchini, cut into 1•inch slices
• 1 red onion, cut into 1•inch pieces
• 2 tbsp olive oil
• 1 tsp dried oregano
• 1 tsp garlic powder
• Salt and pepper to taste
• Wooden or metal skewers

Instructions:

1. If using wooden skewers, soak them in water for 30 minutes to prevent them from burning.

2. In a large bowl, combine the cubed chicken, bell pepper, zucchini, and red onion.

3. Drizzle the olive oil over the chicken and vegetables, and then sprinkle with the dried oregano, garlic powder, salt, and pepper. Toss everything together until the ingredients are evenly coated.

4. Thread the chicken and vegetables onto the skewers, alternating the ingredients.

5. Preheat your grill or grill pan to medium•high heat.

6. Grill the skewers for 12•15 minutes, turning occasionally, until the chicken is cooked through and the vegetables are tender.

7. Serve the Chicken and Vegetable Skewers hot, with any desired dipping sauces or toppings.

Tips for young chefs:
• Let them help cut the chicken and vegetables into the appropriate sizes.
• Encourage them to toss the ingredients with the oil and seasonings.
• Have them carefully thread the chicken and veggies onto the skewers.
• Assist them in safely placing the skewers on the hot grill or grill pan.

These Chicken and Vegetable Skewers are a fun and healthy meal that kids can enjoy making and eating. The combination of juicy chicken and fresh vegetables makes for a delicious and balanced dish.

23. Tuna Salad Sandwich

Ingredient:

• 1 (5 oz) can of tuna, drained
• 2 tbsp mayonnaise
• 1 tbsp diced celery
• 1 tbsp diced onion (optional)
• 1 tsp lemon juice
• Salt and pepper to taste
• 2 slices of bread (whole wheat, white, or your favorite)
• Lettuce leaves (optional)
• Tomato slices (optional)

Instructions:

1. In a small bowl, combine the drained tuna, mayonnaise, diced celery, diced onion (if using), and lemon juice. Mix everything together until well combined.

2. Season the tuna salad with a pinch of salt and pepper to taste.

3. Place one slice of bread on a clean surface. Scoop the tuna salad onto the bread and spread it evenly.

4. If desired, top the tuna salad with lettuce leaves and tomato slices.

5. Place the second slice of bread on top to create a sandwich.

6. Cut the sandwich in half, if desired, and serve.

Tips for young chefs:
• Let them help drain the tuna and mix the tuna salad ingredients.
• Encourage them to season the tuna salad with salt and pepper.
• Have them assemble the sandwich by spreading the tuna salad and adding any desired toppings.
• Allow them to cut the sandwich in half, if they'd like.

This Tuna Salad Sandwich is a classic and nutritious lunch option that's easy for kids to make. The combination of flavorful tuna, creamy mayonnaise, and crunchy vegetables makes it a satisfying and delicious meal.

24. Lentil Soup

Ingredient:

• 1 cup dried brown or green lentils, rinsed
• 4 cups vegetable or chicken broth
• 1 onion, diced
• 2 carrots, peeled and diced
• 2 celery stalks, diced
• 3 garlic cloves, minced
• 1 tsp ground cumin
• 1 tsp dried thyme
• Salt and pepper to taste
• Chopped parsley or cilantro for garnish (optional)

Instructions:

1. In a large pot, combine the rinsed lentils and broth. Bring to a boil over high heat.

2. Once boiling, reduce heat to medium•low and let the lentils simmer for 15•20 minutes, until tender.

3. While the lentils are simmering, sauté the onion, carrots, celery, and garlic in a skillet with a bit of oil over medium heat for 5•7 minutes, until softened.

4. Add the sautéed vegetables, cumin, and thyme to the pot with the lentils. Stir to combine.

5. Season with salt and pepper to taste.

6. Serve the lentil soup hot, garnished with chopped parsley or cilantro if desired.

Tips for Young Chefs:
• Have kids help measure and rinse the lentils.
• Let them practice their chopping skills on the vegetables.
• Encourage them to smell and taste the different spices.
• Discuss the importance of tasting and adjusting seasoning as needed.
• Talk about food safety, such as washing hands and using clean utensils.

This Lentil Soup is a nutritious, flavorful, and easy•to•make dish that's perfect for young chefs to try. The simple ingredients and straightforward preparation make it a great recipe for kids to learn. Enjoy!

25. Caprese Salad

Ingredient:

- 8 oz fresh mozzarella cheese, sliced
- 2 medium tomatoes, sliced
- 8·10 fresh basil leaves
- 2 tbsp extra·virgin olive oil
- 1 tbsp balsamic glaze or reduction
- Salt and pepper to taste

Instructions:

1. Arrange the sliced mozzarella and tomatoes on a serving plate or platter in an overlapping pattern.

2. Gently tear or chiffonade the fresh basil leaves and sprinkle them over the mozzarella and tomatoes.

3. Drizzle the olive oil and balsamic glaze over the salad.

4. Season with salt and pepper to taste.

Tips for Young Chefs:

- Have kids help arrange the mozzarella and tomato slices in a pretty pattern.

- Teach them how to tear or chiffonade the basil leaves (rolling them up and slicing thinly).

- Encourage them to drizzle the olive oil and balsamic glaze artfully over the salad.

- Discuss the importance of using fresh, high·quality ingredients for the best flavor.

- Talk about food safety, such as washing hands and using clean utensils.

This Caprese Salad is a simple, fresh, and delicious dish that's perfect for young chefs to make. It's a great way to introduce them to the concept of using seasonal, quality ingredients to create a beautiful and tasty salad. Enjoy!

26. BLT Sandwich

Ingredient:

• 8 slices bacon
• 4 slices bread (white, whole wheat, or sourdough)
• 2 tomatoes, sliced
• 4 leaves lettuce (such as romaine or iceberg)
• Mayonnaise (optional)
• Salt and pepper to taste

Instructions:

1. Cook the bacon in a skillet or on a baking sheet until crispy. Drain on paper towels.

2. Toast the bread slices until lightly golden brown.

3. Spread a thin layer of mayonnaise on one side of each slice of toast, if desired.

4. Layer the BLT ingredients on the toast in this order:
   • 2 slices of bacon
   • 2•3 tomato slices
   • 2 lettuce leaves

5. Top with the remaining slices of toast.

6. Cut the sandwiches in half diagonally, if desired.

7. Serve immediately.

Tips for Young Chefs:
• Have an adult help with cooking the bacon, as it can splatter.
• Encourage kids to help assemble the sandwiches, layering the ingredients.
• Suggest adding other toppings like avocado or cheese, if desired.
• Discuss food safety, such as washing hands and using clean utensils.

This classic BLT sandwich is a great option for young chefs to make. It's simple, delicious, and allows them to practice their sandwich•making skills. Enjoy!

27. Stuffed Bell Peppers

Ingredient:

• 4 bell peppers (any color)
• 1 lb ground turkey or ground beef
• 1 cup cooked rice
• 1 small onion, diced
• 2 cloves garlic, minced
• 1 can (14.5 oz) diced tomatoes
• 1 tsp dried oregano
• 1 tsp dried basil
• Salt and pepper to taste
• 1 cup shredded cheese (cheddar, mozzarella, or a blend)

Instructions:

1. Preheat the oven to 375°F.

2. Cut the tops off the bell peppers and remove the seeds and membranes. Place the peppers in a baking dish.

3. In a skillet, cook the ground turkey or beef over medium heat until browned and crumbled, about 5•7 minutes. Drain any excess fat.

4. Add the onion and garlic to the skillet and cook for 2•3 minutes until softened.

5. Stir in the cooked rice, diced tomatoes, oregano, basil, salt, and pepper. Mix well.

6. Spoon the meat and rice mixture into the hollowed•out bell peppers, packing it in firmly.

7. Top each stuffed pepper with shredded cheese.

8. Bake for 25•30 minutes, until the peppers are tender and the cheese is melted and bubbly. Serve the stuffed peppers hot.

This Stuffed Bell Pepper recipe is a great way to get young chefs involved in the kitchen. The colorful peppers and flavorful filling make for a delicious and nutritious meal. Enjoy!

28. Veggie Burger

Ingredient:

• 1 (15 oz) can black beans, drained and rinsed
• 1 cup cooked brown rice
• 1/2 cup rolled oats
• 1/2 cup grated carrot
• 1/4 cup finely chopped onion
• 2 cloves garlic, minced
• 1 tsp chili powder
• 1 tsp cumin
• 1/2 tsp salt
• 1/4 tsp black pepper
• Burger buns or lettuce wraps
• Desired toppings (lettuce, tomato, avocado, etc.)

Instructions:

1. In a large bowl, mash the black beans with a fork or potato masher until slightly chunky.

2. Add the cooked rice, rolled oats, grated carrot, onion, garlic, chili powder, cumin, salt, and pepper. Mix well until fully combined.

3. Divide the mixture into 4•6 equal portions and shape them into patties, about 1/2 inch thick.

4. Heat a large skillet or griddle over medium heat. Cook the veggie patties for 3•4 minutes per side, until lightly browned and heated through.

5. Serve the veggie burgers on buns or lettuce wraps, topped with your desired toppings.

Tips for Young Chefs:
• Have kids help mash the black beans and mix the ingredients together.
• Let them practice shaping the patties and cooking them in the skillet.
• Encourage them to get creative with the toppings they want to add.
• Discuss the importance of food safety, such as washing hands and using clean utensils.

These homemade Veggie Burgers are a great option for young chefs to make. They're packed with wholesome ingredients, easy to prepare, and customizable to individual tastes. Enjoy your delicious veggie burgers!

29. Chicken Fajitas

Ingredient:

• 1 lb boneless, skinless chicken breasts, sliced into thin strips
• 1 red bell pepper, sliced into strips
• 1 green bell pepper, sliced into strips
• 1 onion, sliced into strips
• 2 tbsp olive oil
• 1 tbsp fajita seasoning (or make your own with chili powder, cumin, garlic powder, etc.)
• 8•10 small flour or corn tortillas
• Toppings: shredded cheese, sour cream, salsa, guacamole (optional)

Instructions:

1. In a large skillet or wok, heat the olive oil over medium•high heat.

2. Add the chicken strips and fajita seasoning. Cook for 5•7 minutes, stirring occasionally, until the chicken is cooked through.

3. Add the sliced bell peppers and onions to the skillet. Cook for 5•7 more minutes, until the vegetables are tender•crisp.

4. Remove the skillet from heat.

5. Warm the tortillas according to package instructions.

6. To serve, let everyone assemble their own fajitas by placing some of the chicken and veggie mixture into a tortilla. Top with desired toppings like cheese, sour cream, salsa, etc.

This is a fun, interactive meal that kids can customize to their liking. The prep work of slicing the chicken and veggies is great for young chefs to help with. Enjoy your homemade chicken fajitas!

30. Zucchini Noodles with Pesto

Ingredient:

• 3 medium zucchinis, spiralized or julienned into noodles
• 1/2 cup basil pesto (store•bought or homemade)
• 1/4 cup cherry tomatoes, halved
• 2 tbsp toasted pine nuts or sliced almonds
• Grated Parmesan cheese (optional)
• Salt and pepper to taste

Instructions:

1. Using a spiralizer, julienne slicer, or vegetable peeler, cut the zucchinis into long, thin noodle•like strips.

2. In a large bowl, toss the zucchini noodles with the basil pesto until the noodles are evenly coated.

3. Add the halved cherry tomatoes and toasted pine nuts or almonds. Gently mix to combine.

4. Season with salt and pepper to taste.

5. Serve the zucchini noodles with pesto immediately, optionally topped with a sprinkle of grated Parmesan cheese.

Tips for Young Chefs:
• Have kids help spiralize or julienne the zucchinis into noodles. This is a fun, hands•on task.

• Let them assist with mixing the pesto into the zucchini noodles.

• Encourage them to add the tomatoes and nuts, and to taste and season the dish.

• Discuss the benefits of using fresh, healthy ingredients like zucchini and basil.

• Talk about food safety, such as washing hands and using clean utensils.

This Zucchini Noodles with Pesto dish is a great way to introduce young chefs to the concept of "zoodles" (zucchini noodles) and the versatility of pesto. It's a simple, nutritious, and delicious meal that kids will enjoy making and eating. Enjoy!

31. Grilled Salmon with Asparagus

Ingredient:

- 4 salmon fillets (about 4•6 oz each)
- 1 lb asparagus, trimmed
- 2 tbsp olive oil
- 1 tsp lemon juice
- Salt and pepper to taste

Instructions:

1. Preheat grill or grill pan to medium•high heat.

2. In a large bowl, toss the asparagus with 1 tbsp of the olive oil, salt, and pepper.

3. Place the salmon fillets on a plate and brush the tops with the remaining 1 tbsp olive oil. Season with salt and pepper.

4. Grill the salmon for 4•6 minutes per side, until it flakes easily with a fork.

5. Grill the asparagus for 5•7 minutes, turning occasionally, until tender•crisp.

6. Drizzle the lemon juice over the grilled salmon and asparagus.

7. Serve the salmon and asparagus immediately. Enjoy!

This is a simple, healthy, and delicious meal that young chefs can easily prepare with some adult supervision. The grilled salmon and asparagus make a great pairing.

32. Chicken Parmesan

Ingredient:

- 4 boneless, skinless chicken breasts
- 1 cup all•purpose flour
- 2 eggs, beaten
- 1 cup breadcrumbs
- 1/2 cup grated Parmesan cheese
- 1 tsp dried oregano
- 1/2 tsp garlic powder
- Salt and pepper to taste
- 1 jar (24 oz) marinara sauce
- 1 cup shredded mozzarella cheese

Instructions:

1. Preheat your oven to 400°F.

2. Pound the chicken breasts between two sheets of plastic wrap or wax paper to an even thickness, about 1/2 inch.

3. Set up three shallow dishes: one with the flour, one with the beaten eggs, and one with the breadcrumbs, Parmesan, oregano, garlic powder, salt, and pepper mixed together.

4. Dredge the chicken breasts in the flour, dip them in the egg, and then coat them in the breadcrumb mixture, pressing to adhere.

5. Place the breaded chicken in a baking dish or on a baking sheet lined with parchment paper.

6. Bake the chicken for 20•25 minutes, until golden brown and cooked through.

7. Pour the marinara sauce over the chicken and top with the shredded mozzarella cheese.

8. Return the dish to the oven and bake for an additional 10•15 minutes, until the cheese is melted and bubbly. Serve the Chicken Parmesan hot, with your choice of pasta or a side salad.

This Chicken Parmesan is a classic, family•friendly dish that young chefs will enjoy making and eating. The crispy breaded chicken topped with marinara and melted cheese is a delicious and satisfying meal. Enjoy!

33. Beef Stir·Fry

Ingredient:

- 1 lb beef sirloin or flank steak, thinly sliced
- 2 tbsp vegetable or sesame oil
- 2 cloves garlic, minced
- 1 inch piece fresh ginger, peeled and grated
- 1 red bell pepper, sliced
- 1 cup broccoli florets
- 1 cup sliced mushrooms
- 2 tbsp soy sauce
- 1 tbsp rice vinegar or lime juice
- 1 tsp cornstarch
- Salt and pepper to taste
- Cooked rice or noodles, for serving

Instructions:

1. In a small bowl, mix together the soy sauce, rice vinegar, and cornstarch. Set aside.

2. Heat the oil in a large skillet or wok over high heat.

3. Add the beef and stir·fry for 2·3 minutes until lightly browned. Remove the beef from the skillet and set aside.

4. Add the garlic and ginger to the skillet and cook for 1 minute, until fragrant.

5. Add the bell pepper, broccoli, and mushrooms to the skillet. Stir·fry for 3·4 minutes until the vegetables are tender·crisp.

6. Return the beef to the skillet and pour in the soy sauce mixture. Toss everything together and cook for 1·2 minutes until the sauce has thickened.

7. Season with salt and pepper to taste.

8. Serve the beef stir·fry immediately over cooked rice or noodles.

This Beef Stir·Fry is a quick, healthy, and delicious meal that young chefs will enjoy making and eating. The combination of tender beef and crisp vegetables makes it a family·friendly dish. Enjoy!

34. Shrimp Tacos

Ingredient:

• 1 lb shrimp, peeled and deveined
• 2 tbsp olive oil
• 1 tsp chili powder
• 1 tsp cumin
• 1/2 tsp garlic powder
• Salt and pepper to taste
• 8•10 small corn or flour tortillas
• 1 cup shredded cabbage or coleslaw mix
• 1 avocado, diced
• 1/4 cup crumbled feta or queso fresco
• Lime wedges for serving

For the Creamy Cilantro Sauce:
• 1/2 cup sour cream or plain Greek yogurt
• 1/4 cup chopped fresh cilantro
• 1 tbsp lime juice
• 1 garlic clove, minced
• Salt and pepper to taste

Instructions:

1. In a medium bowl, toss the shrimp with the olive oil, chili powder, cumin, garlic powder, salt, and pepper.

2. Heat a large skillet or grill pan over medium•high heat. Cook the shrimp for 2•3 minutes per side, until opaque and cooked through.

3. In a small bowl, mix together the ingredients for the creamy cilantro sauce.

4. Warm the tortillas according to package instructions.

5. To assemble the tacos, place some of the cooked shrimp in each tortilla. Top with shredded cabbage, diced avocado, and crumbled feta or queso fresco.

6. Drizzle the creamy cilantro sauce over the top. Serve the shrimp tacos immediately with lime wedges on the side.

These Shrimp Tacos are a delicious and easy•to•make meal that young chefs will love. The combination of tender shrimp, fresh veggies, and creamy sauce makes for a flavorful and satisfying taco. Enjoy!

35. Spaghetti Bolognese

Ingredient:

- 1 lb ground beef or ground turkey
- 1 onion, diced
- 2 carrots, peeled and diced
- 2 celery stalks, diced
- 3 cloves garlic, minced
- 1 can (28 oz) crushed tomatoes
- 1 can (6 oz) tomato paste
- 1 cup beef or chicken broth
- 2 tsp dried oregano
- 1 tsp dried basil
- Salt and pepper to taste
- 12 oz spaghetti pasta
- Grated Parmesan cheese for serving (optional)

Instructions:

1. In a large skillet or Dutch oven, cook the ground beef or turkey over medium•high heat until browned and crumbled, 5•7 minutes. Drain any excess fat.

2. Add the diced onion, carrots, celery, and minced garlic to the skillet. Cook for 5•7 minutes, stirring occasionally, until the vegetables are softened.

3. Stir in the crushed tomatoes, tomato paste, broth, oregano, and basil. Season with salt and pepper to taste.

4. Bring the Bolognese sauce to a simmer and let it cook for 20•25 minutes, stirring occasionally, until thickened.

5. While the sauce is simmering, cook the spaghetti according to package instructions. Drain and set aside.

6. Serve the Bolognese sauce over the cooked spaghetti. Sprinkle with grated Parmesan cheese, if desired.

Tips for Young Chefs:
- Have kids help measure and add the ingredients to the skillet.
- Let them practice their chopping skills on the onion, carrots, and celery.
- Encourage them to smell the different herbs and spices.
- Discuss the importance of tasting and adjusting seasoning as needed.
- Talk about food safety, such as washing hands and using clean utensils.

36. Vegetarian Chili

Ingredient:

• 2 tablespoons olive oil
• 1 onion, diced
• 3 cloves garlic, minced
• 2 bell peppers, diced
• 2 cans (15 oz each) black beans, drained and rinsed
• 2 cans (15 oz each) kidney beans, drained and rinsed
• 1 can (28 oz) diced tomatoes
• 2 tablespoons chili powder
• 1 tablespoon ground cumin
• 1 teaspoon dried oregano
• 1 teaspoon salt
• 1/2 teaspoon black pepper
• Shredded cheese, sour cream, and chopped cilantro for serving (optional)

Instructions:

1. In a large pot or Dutch oven, heat the olive oil over medium heat.

2. Add the diced onion and sauté for 5 minutes until translucent.

3. Stir in the minced garlic and diced bell peppers. Cook for 3•4 minutes.

4. Add the black beans, kidney beans, diced tomatoes, chili powder, cumin, oregano, salt, and pepper. Stir to combine.

5. Bring the chili to a simmer and let it cook for 20•25 minutes, stirring occasionally, until the flavors have melded and the chili has thickened.

6. Serve the vegetarian chili hot, topped with shredded cheese, sour cream, and chopped cilantro if desired.

Tips for Young Chefs:
• Have kids help measure and add the ingredients to the pot.
• Let them practice their chopping skills on the onion, peppers, and cilantro.
• Encourage them to smell and taste the different spices.
• Discuss the importance of tasting and adjusting seasoning as needed.
• Talk about food safety, such as washing hands and using clean utensils.

This hearty Vegetarian Chili is a great recipe for young chefs to try. It's packed with protein•rich beans, fresh vegetables, and bold flavors. Enjoy!

37. Chicken Alfredo Pasta

Ingredient:

• 8 oz fettuccine or linguine pasta
• 2 boneless, skinless chicken breasts
• 2 tbsp olive oil
• 1/2 cup heavy cream
• 1/2 cup grated Parmesan cheese
• 2 cloves garlic, minced
• 2 tbsp unsalted butter
• Salt and pepper to taste
• Chopped parsley for garnish (optional)

Instructions:

1. Bring a large pot of salted water to a boil. Cook the pasta according to package instructions until al dente. Drain and set aside.

2. Season the chicken breasts with salt and pepper. Heat the olive oil in a skillet over medium•high heat. Cook the chicken for 5•7 minutes per side, until cooked through. Let the chicken rest for 5 minutes, then slice or shred it.

3. In the same skillet, melt the butter over medium heat. Add the minced garlic and cook for 1 minute, until fragrant.

4. Pour in the heavy cream and whisk in the Parmesan cheese. Bring the sauce to a gentle simmer and cook for 2•3 minutes, stirring frequently, until thickened.

5. Add the cooked pasta and sliced or shredded chicken to the Alfredo sauce. Toss everything together until the pasta is evenly coated.

6. Serve the Chicken Alfredo Pasta hot, garnished with chopped parsley if desired.

Tips for Young Chefs:
• Have kids help measure and add the ingredients to the skillet.
• Let them practice their chicken slicing or shredding skills.
• Encourage them to smell the garlic as it cooks.
• Discuss the importance of food safety, such as washing hands and using clean utensils.

This creamy Chicken Alfredo Pasta is a classic, comforting dish that young chefs will love. The combination of tender chicken, rich Alfredo sauce, and al dente pasta makes for a delicious and satisfying meal. Enjoy!

38. Baked Lemon Chicken

Ingredient:

- 4 boneless, skinless chicken breasts
- 2 tablespoons olive oil
- 2 tablespoons lemon juice
- 2 cloves garlic, minced
- 1 teaspoon dried oregano
- 1/2 teaspoon salt
- 1/4 teaspoon black pepper
- 1 lemon, sliced (optional)

Instructions:

1. Preheat your oven to 400°F.

2. In a shallow baking dish, arrange the chicken breasts in a single layer.

3. In a small bowl, whisk together the olive oil, lemon juice, minced garlic, oregano, salt, and pepper.

4. Pour the lemon•garlic mixture over the chicken, making sure to coat the chicken evenly.

5. If desired, arrange lemon slices around the chicken in the baking dish.

6. Bake the chicken for 25•30 minutes, or until it is cooked through and the juices run clear.

7. Remove the chicken from the oven and let it rest for a few minutes before serving.

Tips for Young Chefs:
- Have kids help measure and mix the lemon•garlic marinade.
- Let them arrange the chicken and lemon slices in the baking dish.
- Encourage them to smell the different herbs and spices.
- Discuss the importance of food safety, such as washing hands and using clean utensils.

This Baked Lemon Chicken is a simple, flavorful dish that's perfect for young chefs to make. The bright lemon and garlic flavors complement the tender chicken perfectly. Serve it with your choice of sides for a delicious and healthy meal. Enjoy!

39. Pork Tenderloin with Roasted Vegetables

Ingredient:

• 1 lb pork tenderloin
• 2 tbsp olive oil, divided
• 1 tsp dried thyme
• 1 tsp garlic powder
• Salt and pepper to taste
• 1 lb mixed vegetables (such as potatoes, carrots, Brussels sprouts, onions), cut into 1•inch pieces
• 2 cloves garlic, minced

Instructions:

1. Preheat your oven to 400°F.

2. In a small bowl, mix together 1 tbsp of the olive oil, the dried thyme, garlic powder, and a pinch of salt and pepper. Rub this seasoning mixture all over the pork tenderloin.

3. Place the pork tenderloin in a baking dish or on a rimmed baking sheet.

4. In a large bowl, toss the chopped vegetables with the remaining 1 tbsp of olive oil, minced garlic, and a sprinkle of salt and pepper.

5. Arrange the seasoned vegetables around the pork tenderloin in the baking dish or on the baking sheet.

6. Roast the pork and vegetables in the preheated oven for 25•30 minutes, or until the pork reaches an internal temperature of 145°F and the vegetables are tender.

7. Remove the pork and vegetables from the oven and let the pork rest for 5 minutes before slicing. Slice the pork tenderloin and serve it with the roasted vegetables.

Tips for Young Chefs:
• Have kids help measure and mix the seasoning for the pork.
• Let them practice their vegetable chopping skills.
• Encourage them to smell the herbs and garlic as they cook.
• Discuss the importance of food safety, such as washing hands and using clean utensils.

40. Veggie Pizza

Ingredient:

• 1 pre•made pizza crust or dough
• 1/2 cup pizza sauce
• 1 cup shredded mozzarella cheese
• 1/2 cup sliced mushrooms
• 1/2 cup diced bell peppers
• 1/2 cup diced onions
• 1/2 cup sliced black olives (optional)
• 1 tsp dried oregano
• Salt and pepper to taste

Instructions:

1. Preheat your oven to 425°F.

2. If using pre•made dough, roll or stretch it out to fit your pizza pan or baking sheet. If using a pre•made crust, skip this step.

3. Spread the pizza sauce evenly over the crust.

4. Sprinkle the shredded mozzarella cheese over the sauce.

5. Arrange the sliced mushrooms, diced bell peppers, and diced onions over the cheese.

6. If using, scatter the sliced black olives over the top.

7. Sprinkle the dried oregano over the entire pizza, and season with a pinch of salt and pepper.

8. Bake the pizza for 12•15 minutes, or until the crust is golden brown and the cheese is melted and bubbly.

9. Remove the pizza from the oven and let it cool for a few minutes before slicing and serving.

This Veggie Pizza is a great way to get young chefs involved in the kitchen. It's a healthy and delicious option that allows them to customize the toppings to their liking. Enjoy your homemade veggie pizza!

41. Stuffed Portobello Mushrooms

Ingredient:

• 4 large portobello mushroom caps, stems removed and chopped
• 2 tbsp olive oil
• 1/2 cup diced onion
• 2 cloves garlic, minced
• 1/2 cup diced bell pepper
• 1 cup cooked quinoa or brown rice
• 1/2 cup shredded mozzarella cheese
• 2 tbsp grated Parmesan cheese
• 1 tsp dried oregano
• Salt and pepper to taste

Instructions:

1. Preheat your oven to 400°F.

2. Gently clean the portobello mushroom caps with a damp paper towel. Remove and chop the stems.

3. In a skillet, heat the olive oil over medium heat. Add the chopped mushroom stems, diced onion, and minced garlic. Sauté for 3•4 minutes until softened.

4. Stir in the diced bell pepper and cook for another 2•3 minutes.

5. Remove the skillet from heat and stir in the cooked quinoa or brown rice, mozzarella cheese, Parmesan cheese, and dried oregano. Season with salt and pepper to taste.

6. Arrange the portobello mushroom caps, gill•side up, on a baking sheet. Spoon the stuffing mixture evenly into the mushroom caps.

7. Bake the stuffed mushrooms for 15•20 minutes, until the mushrooms are tender and the cheese is melted and bubbly.

8. Serve the stuffed portobello mushrooms warm.

These Stuffed Portobello Mushrooms are a delicious and healthy vegetarian option that young chefs can easily prepare. The combination of savory fillings and tender mushrooms makes for a satisfying and flavorful dish. Enjoy!

42. Fish Tacos

Ingredient:

• 1 lb white fish fillets (such as tilapia, cod, or halibut), cut into 1•inch pieces
• 2 tbsp olive oil
• 1 tsp chili powder
• 1 tsp cumin
• 1/2 tsp garlic powder
• Salt and pepper to taste
• 8•10 small corn or flour tortillas
• 2 cups shredded cabbage or coleslaw mix
• 1 avocado, diced
• 1/4 cup crumbled feta or queso fresco
• Lime wedges for serving

For the Creamy Cilantro Sauce:
• 1/2 cup sour cream or plain Greek yogurt
• 1/4 cup chopped fresh cilantro
• 1 tbsp lime juice
• 1 garlic clove, minced
• Salt and pepper to taste

Instructions:

1. In a medium bowl, toss the fish pieces with the olive oil, chili powder, cumin, garlic powder, salt, and pepper.

2. Heat a large skillet or grill pan over medium•high heat. Cook the fish for 2•3 minutes per side, until opaque and cooked through.

3. In a small bowl, mix together the ingredients for the creamy cilantro sauce.

4. Warm the tortillas according to package instructions.

5. To assemble the tacos, place some of the cooked fish in each tortilla. Top with shredded cabbage, diced avocado, and crumbled feta or queso fresco.

6. Drizzle the creamy cilantro sauce over the top. Serve the fish tacos immediately with lime wedges on the side.

These Fish Tacos are a delicious and easy•to•make meal that young chefs will love. The flaky white fish, fresh veggies, and creamy sauce make for a flavorful and satisfying taco. Enjoy!

43. Chicken and Broccoli Stir·Fry

Ingredient:

- 1 lb boneless, skinless chicken breasts, cut into 1·inch pieces
- 2 tbsp vegetable or sesame oil
- 3 cups broccoli florets
- 1 red bell pepper, sliced
- 3 cloves garlic, minced
- 1 tbsp grated fresh ginger
- 2 tbsp soy sauce
- 1 tbsp rice vinegar or lime juice
- 1 tsp cornstarch
- Salt and pepper to taste
- Cooked rice or noodles, for serving

Instructions:

1. In a small bowl, whisk together the soy sauce, rice vinegar, and cornstarch. Set aside.

2. Heat the oil in a large skillet or wok over high heat.

3. Add the chicken to the hot skillet and stir·fry for 3·4 minutes, until the chicken is lightly browned.

4. Add the broccoli florets and sliced bell pepper to the skillet. Stir·fry for 3·4 minutes, until the vegetables are tender·crisp.

5. Stir in the minced garlic and grated ginger. Cook for 1 minute, until fragrant.

6. Pour the soy sauce mixture into the skillet and toss everything together. Cook for 1·2 minutes, until the sauce has thickened.

7. Season the stir·fry with salt and pepper to taste. Serve the Chicken and Broccoli Stir·Fry immediately over cooked rice or noodles.

Tips for Young Chefs:
- Have kids help measure and prepare the ingredients.
- Let them practice their chopping and slicing skills on the vegetables.
- Encourage them to smell the garlic and ginger as they cook.
- Discuss the importance of food safety, such as washing hands and using clean utensils.

44. Baked Ziti

Ingredient:

• 12 oz ziti pasta or other short, tubular pasta
• 1 lb ground beef or Italian sausage (optional)
• 1 onion, diced
• 3 cloves garlic, minced
• 1 jar (24•28 oz) marinara sauce
• 1 cup ricotta cheese
• 1 egg
• 1/2 cup grated Parmesan cheese
• 2 cups shredded mozzarella cheese
• Salt and pepper to taste

Instructions:

1. Preheat the oven to 375°F.

2. Cook the ziti according to package instructions until al dente. Drain and set aside.

3. If using ground beef or sausage, cook it in a skillet over medium heat until browned and crumbled. Drain any excess fat.

4. Add the diced onion and minced garlic to the skillet. Cook for 2•3 minutes until softened.

5. Stir in the marinara sauce and simmer for 5 minutes.

6. In a separate bowl, mix together the ricotta cheese, egg, and 1/4 cup of the Parmesan cheese.

7. In a 9x13 inch baking dish, layer half of the cooked ziti, half of the ricotta mixture, half of the meat sauce, and 1 cup of the mozzarella cheese.

8. Repeat the layers, ending with the remaining mozzarella cheese and Parmesan cheese.

9. Bake for 25•30 minutes, until the cheese is melted and bubbly. Let the baked ziti cool for 5•10 minutes before serving.

This Baked Ziti is a classic, comforting dish that's perfect for young chefs to make. The layers of pasta, cheese, and sauce make it a crowd•pleaser. Enjoy!

45. Mushroom Risotto

Ingredient:

• 4 cups low•sodium chicken or vegetable broth
• 2 tbsp olive oil
• 8 oz cremini or button mushrooms, sliced
• 1 onion, diced
• 2 cloves garlic, minced
• 1 cup Arborio rice
• 1/2 cup dry white wine (or additional broth)
• 1/2 cup grated Parmesan cheese
• 2 tbsp unsalted butter
• 2 tbsp chopped fresh parsley
• Salt and pepper to taste

Instructions:

1. In a saucepan, bring the broth to a simmer over medium heat. Reduce heat to low to keep the broth warm.

2. In a large skillet, heat the olive oil over medium•high heat. Add the sliced mushrooms and sauté for 5•7 minutes, until they are lightly browned. Remove the mushrooms from the skillet and set aside.

3. In the same skillet, sauté the diced onion for 3•4 minutes until translucent. Add the minced garlic and cook for 1 minute more.

4. Add the Arborio rice to the skillet and stir to coat the grains with the oil. Cook for 2•3 minutes, until the rice is lightly toasted.

5. Pour in the white wine (or additional broth) and stir constantly until the liquid is absorbed, about 2•3 minutes.

6. Ladle in about 1/2 cup of the warm broth and stir continuously until the liquid is absorbed. Continue this process, adding 1/2 cup of broth at a time, until the rice is tender and creamy, about 20•25 minutes total.

7. Stir in the sautéed mushrooms, Parmesan cheese, and butter until well combined.

8. Remove from heat and stir in the chopped parsley. Season with salt and pepper to taste.Serve the Mushroom Risotto immediately.

46. Chicken and Rice Casserole

Ingredient:

• 1 lb boneless, skinless chicken breasts, cut into 1•inch pieces
• 1 cup uncooked long•grain white rice
• 1 can (10.5 oz) cream of mushroom soup
• 1 can (10.5 oz) cream of chicken soup
• 1 cup milk
• 1 cup frozen peas
• 1/2 cup shredded cheddar cheese
• 1 tsp dried thyme
• Salt and pepper to taste

Instructions:

1. Preheat your oven to 375°F.

2. In a large bowl, combine the cubed chicken, uncooked rice, cream of mushroom soup, cream of chicken soup, milk, frozen peas, shredded cheddar, and dried thyme. Stir until well mixed.

3. Transfer the chicken and rice mixture to a 9x13 inch baking dish. Spread it out evenly.

4. Cover the baking dish with aluminum foil and bake for 45•55 minutes, until the rice is tender and the chicken is cooked through.

5. Remove the foil and bake for an additional 10•15 minutes, until the top is lightly browned. Let the casserole cool for 5•10 minutes before serving.

Tips for Young Chefs:
• Have kids help measure and add the ingredients to the mixing bowl.
• Let them practice their stirring skills to combine everything well.
• Encourage them to smell the herbs and spices as they cook.
• Discuss the importance of food safety, such as washing hands and using clean utensils.

This Chicken and Rice Casserole is a comforting, one•dish meal that young chefs can easily prepare. The combination of tender chicken, fluffy rice, and creamy sauces makes it a family•friendly dish. Serve it with a fresh salad for a complete and satisfying dinner. Enjoy!

47. Teriyaki Chicken

Ingredient:

• 1 lb boneless, skinless chicken breasts, cut into 1•inch pieces
• 1/2 cup teriyaki sauce (store•bought or homemade)
• 2 tbsp vegetable or sesame oil
• 2 cloves garlic, minced
• 1 inch piece fresh ginger, peeled and grated
• 1 cup broccoli florets
• 1 red bell pepper, sliced
• 2 cups cooked rice, for serving

Instructions:

1. In a medium bowl, toss the chicken pieces with the teriyaki sauce. Cover and let marinate for 15•30 minutes.

2. Heat the oil in a large skillet or wok over medium•high heat.

3. Add the marinated chicken to the hot skillet and stir•fry for 4•5 minutes, until the chicken is lightly browned.

4. Add the minced garlic and grated ginger to the skillet. Cook for 1 minute, until fragrant.

5. Stir in the broccoli florets and sliced bell pepper. Continue to stir•fry for 3•4 minutes, until the vegetables are tender•crisp.

6. If the sauce seems too thick, you can add a splash of water or chicken broth to thin it out. Serve the Teriyaki Chicken immediately over the cooked rice.

Tips for Young Chefs:
• Have kids help measure and mix the chicken with the teriyaki sauce.
• Let them practice their vegetable chopping skills on the broccoli and bell pepper.
• Encourage them to smell the garlic and ginger as they cook.
• Discuss the importance of food safety, such as washing hands and using clean utensils.

This Teriyaki Chicken is a delicious and easy•to•make dish that young chefs will enjoy. The combination of tender chicken, fresh vegetables, and flavorful teriyaki sauce makes for a satisfying and nutritious meal. Serve it over rice for a complete and balanced dinner. Enjoy!

48. Grilled Lamb Chops

Ingredient:

• 8 lamb chops (about 1•inch thick)
• 2 tbsp olive oil
• 2 tsp dried rosemary
• 1 tsp dried thyme
• 1 tsp garlic powder
• Salt and pepper to taste
• Lemon wedges for serving

Instructions:

1. Preheat your grill or grill pan to medium•high heat.

2. In a small bowl, mix together the olive oil, dried rosemary, dried thyme, garlic powder, and a generous pinch of salt and pepper.

3. Rub the seasoning mixture all over the lamb chops, coating them evenly on both sides.

4. Grill the lamb chops for 3•4 minutes per side, or until they reach the desired level of doneness. (For medium•rare, the internal temperature should reach 130•135ºF.)

5. Transfer the grilled lamb chops to a plate and let them rest for 5 minutes before serving.

6. Serve the lamb chops warm, with lemon wedges on the side.

Tips for Young Chefs:
• Have kids help measure and mix the seasoning ingredients.
• Let them practice brushing the seasoning onto the lamb chops.
• Encourage them to smell the herbs as they cook.
• Discuss the importance of food safety, such as washing hands and using clean utensils.

These Grilled Lamb Chops are a delicious and easy•to•prepare main dish that young chefs will enjoy. The flavorful seasoning and quick cooking time make it a great option for a family meal. Serve the lamb chops with your choice of sides for a complete and satisfying dinner. Enjoy!

49. Beef Tacos

Ingredient:

• 1 lb ground beef
• 1 onion, diced
• 2 cloves garlic, minced
• 1 tbsp chili powder
• 1 tsp ground cumin
• 1 tsp dried oregano
• 1/2 tsp paprika
• Salt and pepper to taste
• 8•10 small corn or flour tortillas
• Shredded lettuce, diced tomatoes, shredded cheese, sour cream, and salsa for serving

Instructions:

1. In a large skillet over medium•high heat, cook the ground beef, breaking it up with a wooden spoon, until browned and cooked through, about 5•7 minutes.

2. Drain any excess fat from the skillet.

3. Add the diced onion and minced garlic to the skillet. Cook for 2•3 minutes, until the onion is translucent.

4. Stir in the chili powder, cumin, oregano, paprika, and a pinch of salt and pepper. Cook for 1•2 minutes to toast the spices.

5. Warm the tortillas according to package instructions.

6. To assemble the tacos, place some of the seasoned ground beef in each tortilla. Top with shredded lettuce, diced tomatoes, shredded cheese, sour cream, and salsa.

7. Serve the beef tacos immediately.

These classic Beef Tacos are a crowd•pleasing and easy•to•make meal that young chefs will love. The flavorful seasoned ground beef, combined with the fresh toppings, makes for a delicious and satisfying taco. Enjoy!

50. Vegetable Lasagna

Ingredient:

• 9 lasagna noodles
• 2 cups ricotta cheese
• 1 egg
• 1/2 cup grated Parmesan cheese
• 1 tsp dried basil
• 1/2 tsp salt
• 1/4 tsp black pepper
• 2 cups shredded mozzarella cheese
• 2 cups chopped vegetables (such as spinach, zucchini, bell peppers, mushrooms)
• 1 jar (24 oz) marinara sauce

Instructions:

1. Preheat your oven to 375°F (190°C).

2. Cook the lasagna noodles according to the package instructions. Drain and set aside.

3. In a medium bowl, mix together the ricotta cheese, egg, Parmesan cheese, basil, salt, and pepper until well combined.

4. Spread 1/2 cup of the marinara sauce in the bottom of a 9x13 inch baking dish.

5. Layer 3 lasagna noodles over the sauce. Spread half of the ricotta cheese mixture over the noodles, then top with half of the chopped vegetables and 1/2 cup of the mozzarella cheese.

6. Repeat the layers of noodles, ricotta cheese, vegetables, and mozzarella cheese.

7. Top with the remaining 3 lasagna noodles and the remaining marinara sauce.

8. Cover the dish with aluminum foil and bake for 30 minutes.

9. Remove the foil and bake for an additional 15 minutes, or until the cheese is melted and bubbly. Let the lasagna cool for 10•15 minutes before serving.

This vegetable lasagna is a great way to get kids to eat their veggies! The layers of noodles, creamy ricotta, and flavorful vegetables make for a delicious and satisfying meal. Enjoy!

51. Honey Glazed Salmon

Ingredient:

- 4 salmon fillets (about 1 lb total)
- 2 tbsp honey
- 1 tbsp soy sauce
- 1 tsp Dijon mustard
- 1 tsp lemon juice
- Salt and pepper to taste

Instructions:

1. Preheat your oven to 400°F (200°C).

2. In a small bowl, whisk together the honey, soy sauce, Dijon mustard, and lemon juice to make the glaze.

3. Season the salmon fillets with salt and pepper on both sides.

4. Place the salmon fillets on a baking sheet lined with parchment paper or foil.

5. Brush the top of the salmon fillets with the honey glaze, making sure to coat them evenly.

6. Bake the salmon in the preheated oven for 12•15 minutes, or until the salmon is cooked through and flakes easily with a fork.

7. Serve the honey glazed salmon immediately, with any extra glaze drizzled over the top.

This recipe is easy to follow and the sweet and savory glaze makes the salmon really delicious. It's a great option for young chefs to try out, as it's simple to prepare but still looks and tastes impressive. Enjoy!

52. BBQ Chicken Pizza

Ingredient:

• 1 pre•made pizza crust or dough
• 1 cup cooked, shredded chicken
• 1/2 cup barbecue sauce
• 1 cup shredded mozzarella cheese
• 1/4 cup sliced red onion
• 2 tbsp chopped fresh cilantro (optional)

Instructions:

1. Preheat your oven to 400°F (200°C).

2. If using pre•made pizza dough, roll or stretch it out to fit your pizza pan or baking sheet.

3. Spread the barbecue sauce evenly over the pizza crust, leaving a small border around the edges.

4. Sprinkle the shredded chicken over the barbecue sauce.

5. Top the chicken with the shredded mozzarella cheese.

6. Arrange the sliced red onions over the cheese.

7. Bake the pizza in the preheated oven for 12•15 minutes, or until the crust is golden brown and the cheese is melted and bubbly.

8. Remove the pizza from the oven and sprinkle the chopped fresh cilantro over the top, if using.

9. Slice the pizza and serve hot.

This BBQ Chicken Pizza is a fun and flavorful twist on a classic pizza. The sweet and tangy barbecue sauce, tender chicken, and melty cheese make for a delicious combination. It's a great recipe for young chefs to try, as it's easy to assemble and bake. Enjoy!

53. Pasta Primavera

Ingredient:

• 8 oz pasta (such as penne, farfalle, or linguine)
• 2 tbsp olive oil
• 1 cup broccoli florets
• 1 cup sliced zucchini
• 1 cup sliced mushrooms
• 1 red bell pepper, sliced
• 2 cloves garlic, minced
• 1/2 cup frozen peas
• 1/4 cup grated Parmesan cheese
• 2 tbsp chopped fresh basil or parsley
• Salt and pepper to taste

For the Lemon Garlic Sauce:
• 1/4 cup olive oil
• 2 tbsp lemon juice
• 2 cloves garlic, minced
• 1 tsp Dijon mustard
• Salt and pepper to taste

Instructions:

1. Bring a large pot of salted water to a boil. Cook the pasta according to package instructions until al dente. Drain and set aside.

2. In a large skillet, heat the 2 tbsp of olive oil over medium•high heat. Add the broccoli, zucchini, mushrooms, and bell pepper. Sauté for 5•7 minutes, until the vegetables are tender•crisp.

3. Add the minced garlic to the skillet and cook for 1 minute, until fragrant.

4. Stir in the cooked pasta, frozen peas, Parmesan cheese, and chopped basil or parsley. Toss to combine.

5. In a small bowl, whisk together the ingredients for the lemon garlic sauce.

6. Pour the lemon garlic sauce over the pasta primavera and toss to coat everything evenly.

7. Season the pasta primavera with salt and pepper to taste.

8. Serve the pasta primavera warm, garnished with additional Parmesan cheese and fresh herbs if desired.

This Pasta Primavera is a colorful, flavorful, and healthy dish that young chefs will enjoy making and eating. The combination of fresh vegetables and the bright lemon garlic sauce makes it a delicious and satisfying meal. Enjoy!

54. Chicken Pot Pie

Ingredient:

- 1 cup chicken broth
- 1 cup milk
- 1 tsp dried thyme
- 1/2 tsp dried rosemary
- Salt and pepper to taste
- 1 (9•inch) refrigerated pie crust

- 1 lb boneless, skinless chicken breasts, cubed
- 2 tbsp olive oil
- 1 onion, diced
- 2 carrots, peeled and diced
- 2 celery stalks, diced
- 2 cloves garlic, minced
- 2 tbsp all•purpose flour

Instructions:

1. Preheat your oven to 400°F (200°C).

2. In a large skillet, heat the olive oil over medium•high heat. Add the cubed chicken and cook until browned, about 5•7 minutes. Remove the chicken from the skillet and set aside.

3. In the same skillet, add the onion, carrots, celery, and garlic. Cook for 5•7 minutes, until the vegetables are softened.

4. Sprinkle the flour over the vegetables and stir to coat. Cook for 2 minutes, stirring constantly.

5. Gradually pour in the chicken broth and milk, whisking constantly to prevent lumps. Bring the mixture to a simmer and cook for 5•7 minutes, until the sauce has thickened.

6. Stir in the cooked chicken, thyme, rosemary, and season with salt and pepper to taste.

7. Transfer the chicken and vegetable mixture to a 9•inch pie dish.

8. Unroll the refrigerated pie crust and place it over the top of the filling, pressing the edges to seal. Cut a few slits in the top of the crust to allow steam to escape.

9. Bake the Chicken Pot Pie in the preheated oven for 30•35 minutes, or until the crust is golden brown and the filling is bubbly. Let the pie cool for 10•15 minutes before serving.

55. Lentil Curry

Ingredient:

- 1 cup dried brown or green lentils, rinsed
- 1 onion, diced
- 2 cloves garlic, minced
- 1 tbsp grated fresh ginger
- 1 tbsp curry powder
- 1 tsp ground cumin
- 1 tsp ground coriander
- 1/2 tsp ground turmeric
- 1/4 tsp cayenne pepper (optional)
- 1 (14 oz) can diced tomatoes
- 1 cup vegetable or chicken broth
- 1 cup coconut milk
- Salt and pepper to taste
- Chopped fresh cilantro for garnish

Instructions:

1. In a large saucepan, combine the rinsed lentils and 3 cups of water. Bring to a boil, then reduce heat and simmer for 15•20 minutes, until the lentils are tender. Drain and set aside.

2. In the same saucepan, heat a drizzle of oil over medium heat. Add the diced onion and sauté for 5•7 minutes, until translucent.

3. Add the minced garlic and grated ginger. Cook for 1 minute, until fragrant.

4. Stir in the curry powder, cumin, coriander, turmeric, and cayenne (if using). Cook for 2 minutes, stirring constantly, to toast the spices.

5. Pour in the diced tomatoes, broth, and coconut milk. Bring the mixture to a simmer.

6. Add the cooked lentils to the saucepan and stir to combine. Simmer for 10•15 minutes, until the sauce has thickened.

7. Season the lentil curry with salt and pepper to taste.

8. Serve the lentil curry over basmati rice or with naan bread. Garnish with chopped fresh cilantro.

This Lentil Curry is a flavorful, vegetarian•friendly dish that's perfect for young chefs to try. The combination of aromatic spices, creamy coconut milk, and hearty lentils makes for a satisfying and nutritious meal. Enjoy!

56. Shrimp Scampi

Ingredient:

- 1 lb large shrimp, peeled and deveined
- 4 tbsp unsalted butter
- 3 cloves garlic, minced
- 1/4 cup dry white wine or chicken broth
- 2 tbsp freshly squeezed lemon juice
- 2 tbsp chopped fresh parsley
- 1/4 tsp red pepper flakes (optional)
- Salt and pepper to taste
- Lemon wedges for serving

Instructions:

1. Rinse the shrimp and pat them dry with paper towels. Set aside.

2. In a large skillet, melt the butter over medium heat. Add the minced garlic and cook for 1•2 minutes, until fragrant.

3. Add the shrimp to the skillet and cook for 2•3 minutes per side, until they start to turn pink and curl up.

4. Pour in the white wine (or chicken broth) and lemon juice. Bring the mixture to a simmer and cook for 2•3 minutes, until the sauce has slightly thickened.

5. Remove the skillet from the heat and stir in the chopped parsley and red pepper flakes (if using). Season with salt and pepper to taste.

6. Serve the shrimp scampi immediately, with lemon wedges on the side. The shrimp can be served over pasta, rice, or with crusty bread to soak up the delicious garlic•lemon sauce.

This Shrimp Scampi is a classic, elegant dish that's easy for young chefs to prepare. The combination of succulent shrimp, garlic, lemon, and butter creates a flavorful and impressive meal. Enjoy!

57. Shepherd's Pie

Ingredient:

- 1 lb ground beef or ground lamb
- 1 onion, diced
- 2 carrots, peeled and diced
- 2 celery stalks, diced
- 2 cloves garlic, minced
- 2 tbsp tomato paste
- 1 tsp dried thyme
- 1 tsp dried rosemary
- 1 cup beef or chicken broth
- 2 tbsp Worcestershire sauce
- Salt and pepper to taste
- 3 cups mashed potatoes (about 4•5 medium potatoes)
- 1 cup shredded cheddar cheese

Instructions:

1. Preheat your oven to 375°F (190°C).

2. In a large skillet or Dutch oven, cook the ground beef or lamb over medium•high heat, breaking it up with a wooden spoon, until browned and cooked through, about 5•7 minutes. Drain any excess fat.

3. Add the onion, carrots, celery, and garlic to the skillet. Cook for 5•7 minutes, until the vegetables are softened.

4. Stir in the tomato paste, thyme, and rosemary. Cook for 2 minutes.

5. Pour in the broth and Worcestershire sauce. Bring the mixture to a simmer and let it cook for 10•15 minutes, until the sauce has thickened.

6. Season the meat mixture with salt and pepper to taste.

7. Spread the meat mixture in an even layer in a 9x13 inch baking dish.

8. Top the meat with the mashed potatoes, spreading them evenly over the top.

9. Sprinkle the shredded cheddar cheese over the mashed potatoes.

10. Bake the Shepherd's Pie in the preheated oven for 25•30 minutes, or until the potatoes are lightly browned and the cheese is melted and bubbly. Let the Shepherd's Pie cool for 5•10 minutes before serving.

This Shepherd's Pie is a comforting and delicious dish that's perfect for young chefs to make. The layers of savory meat, vegetables, and creamy mashed potatoes make it a family•friendly meal. Enjoy!

58. Eggplant Parmesan

Ingredient:

• 2 medium eggplants, sliced into 1/2•inch thick rounds
• 2 eggs, beaten
• 1 cup breadcrumbs
• 1/2 cup grated Parmesan cheese
• 1 tsp dried oregano
• 1/2 tsp garlic powder
• Salt and pepper to taste
• 2 cups marinara sauce
• 2 cups shredded mozzarella cheese

Instructions:

1. Preheat your oven to 375°F (190°C). Grease a 9x13 inch baking dish.

2. In a shallow bowl, beat the eggs. In another shallow bowl, mix together the breadcrumbs, Parmesan cheese, oregano, garlic powder, salt, and pepper.

3. Dip the eggplant slices into the beaten egg, then coat them in the breadcrumb mixture, pressing gently to help it adhere.

4. Arrange the breaded eggplant slices in a single layer in the prepared baking dish.

5. Bake the eggplant for 20 minutes, flipping the slices halfway through, until golden brown.

6. Remove the baked eggplant from the oven and top each slice with a spoonful of marinara sauce.

7. Sprinkle the shredded mozzarella cheese evenly over the top.

8. Return the dish to the oven and bake for an additional 15•20 minutes, or until the cheese is melted and bubbly.

9. Let the Eggplant Parmesan cool for 5•10 minutes before serving.

This Eggplant Parmesan is a delicious and satisfying vegetarian dish that's perfect for young chefs to make. The crispy breaded eggplant, tangy marinara sauce, and melty cheese create a flavorful and comforting meal. Enjoy!

59. Beef and Broccoli

Ingredient:

- 2 cloves garlic, minced
- 1 tsp grated ginger
- 2 tbsp vegetable oil
- 4 cups broccoli florets
- 1/2 cup beef broth
- 1 tbsp cornstarch
- 2 green onions, sliced (optional)
- Cooked rice, for serving

- 1 lb flank steak or sirloin, thinly sliced against the grain
- 2 tbsp soy sauce
- 1 tbsp rice vinegar
- 1 tbsp brown sugar
- 2 tsp sesame oil

Instructions:

1. In a medium bowl, combine the sliced beef, soy sauce, rice vinegar, brown sugar, sesame oil, garlic, and ginger. Toss to coat the beef and let it marinate for 15•20 minutes.

2. In a large skillet or wok, heat the vegetable oil over high heat. Add the broccoli florets and stir•fry for 2•3 minutes, until the broccoli is crisp•tender. Remove the broccoli from the skillet and set aside.

3. Add the marinated beef to the hot skillet and stir•fry for 2•3 minutes, until the beef is mostly cooked through.

4. In a small bowl, whisk together the beef broth and cornstarch until smooth.

5. Pour the beef broth mixture into the skillet with the beef. Bring the sauce to a simmer and cook for 1•2 minutes, until the sauce has thickened.

6. Add the cooked broccoli back to the skillet and toss everything together to coat the broccoli in the sauce.

7. Remove the Beef and Broccoli from the heat and garnish with the sliced green onions, if desired. Serve the Beef and Broccoli immediately over steamed rice.

This Beef and Broccoli is a classic Chinese•American dish that's easy for young chefs to prepare. The tender beef, crisp broccoli, and savory sauce make for a delicious and balanced meal. Enjoy!

60. Chicken Tikka Masala

Ingredient:

• 1 lb boneless, skinless chicken
 breasts, cut into 1•inch cubes
• 1 cup plain yogurt
• 2 tbsp lemon juice
• 2 tsp grated ginger
• 2 tsp grated garlic
• 1 tsp garam masala
• 1 tsp paprika
• 1/2 tsp salt

• 3 cloves garlic, minced
• 1 tbsp grated ginger
• 2 tsp garam masala
• 1 tsp paprika
• 1 tsp ground cumin
• 1/2 tsp cayenne pepper (optional)
• 1 (14 oz) can diced tomatoes
• 1 cup heavy cream
• 1/4 cup chopped fresh cilantro
• Salt and pepper to taste

For the Sauce:
• 2 tbsp oil
• 1 onion, diced

Instructions:

1. In a large bowl, combine the chicken, yogurt, lemon juice, ginger, garlic, garam masala, paprika, and salt. Cover and marinate in the refrigerator for at least 30 minutes (or up to 4 hours).

2. Preheat your oven to 400°F (200°C). Thread the marinated chicken onto skewers and place them on a baking sheet.

3. Bake the chicken for 12•15 minutes, or until cooked through and lightly charred.

4. In a large skillet, heat the oil over medium heat. Add the onion and sauté for 5 minutes, until translucent.

5. Add the garlic, ginger, garam masala, paprika, cumin, and cayenne (if using). Cook for 2 minutes, stirring constantly.

6. Stir in the diced tomatoes and their juices. Simmer for 10 minutes, allowing the flavors to meld.

7. Stir in the heavy cream and the cooked chicken. Simmer for an additional 5 minutes, or until the sauce has thickened.

8. Remove from heat and stir in the chopped cilantro. Season with salt and pepper to taste. Serve the Chicken Tikka Masala over basmati rice or with naan bread

61. Hummus and Veggies

Ingredient:

• 1 (15 oz) can chickpeas (garbanzo beans), drained and rinsed
• 2 tbsp tahini (sesame seed paste)
• 2 tbsp fresh lemon juice
• 1 clove garlic, minced
• 2 tbsp olive oil
• 1/4 tsp ground cumin
• 1/4 tsp paprika
• Salt and pepper to taste
• Assorted fresh vegetables (such as carrot sticks, cucumber slices, bell pepper strips, cherry tomatoes)

Instructions:

1. In a food processor or blender, combine the drained and rinsed chickpeas, tahini, lemon juice, garlic, olive oil, cumin, and paprika. Blend until smooth and creamy, scraping down the sides as needed.

2. Season the hummus with salt and pepper to taste.

3. Transfer the hummus to a serving bowl.

4. Arrange the assorted fresh vegetables around the bowl of hummus, creating a colorful and appetizing presentation.

5. Serve the hummus and veggies immediately, or refrigerate until ready to serve.

This Hummus and Veggies snack is a great option for young chefs because it's easy to make, healthy, and customizable. The creamy, flavorful hummus pairs perfectly with the crunchy, fresh vegetables.

Encourage young chefs to experiment with different vegetable combinations, such as carrot sticks, celery, bell pepper strips, cherry tomatoes, cucumber slices, and more. They can also try adding their own favorite seasonings or toppings to the hummus, like paprika, cumin, or chopped parsley.

Serving the hummus and veggies together as a snack or appetizer is a fun and nutritious way for young chefs to get creative in the kitchen.

62. Apple Slices with Peanut Butter

Ingredient:

• 2 apples, cored and sliced
• 1/2 cup creamy peanut butter
• Optional toppings: honey, cinnamon, raisins, crushed graham crackers

Instructions:

1. Wash the apples and slice them into thin wedges or rounds, removing the core.

2. Arrange the apple slices on a plate or platter.

3. Scoop the peanut butter into a small bowl or dish.

4. Encourage the young chef to dip the apple slices into the peanut butter, coating them evenly.

5. If desired, the chef can drizzle a small amount of honey over the peanut butter•coated apple slices.

6. Sprinkle a pinch of cinnamon over the top, or add any other desired toppings like raisins or crushed graham crackers.

This Apple Slices with Peanut Butter snack is a great option for young chefs because it's:

• Simple to prepare
• Nutritious, with the combination of fruit and protein•rich peanut butter
• Customizable with different toppings
• Fun to assemble and eat

Encourage the young chef to experiment with different types of apples, nut butters (such as almond or cashew butter), and creative toppings. This is a healthy and delicious snack that kids will love making and eating.

63. Trail Mix

Ingredient:

- 1 cup raw almonds
- 1 cup raw cashews
- 1 cup raw pumpkin seeds (pepitas)
- 1 cup dried cranberries
- 1 cup dark chocolate chips or chunks
- 1/2 cup roasted and salted sunflower seeds
- 1/4 cup unsweetened shredded coconut (optional)

Instructions:

1. In a large bowl, combine all the ingredients • the almonds, cashews, pumpkin seeds, dried cranberries, chocolate chips, sunflower seeds, and shredded coconut (if using).

2. Stir the ingredients together until they are evenly mixed.

3. Transfer the trail mix to an airtight container or resealable bag.

4. Store the trail mix at room temperature for up to 2 weeks.

That's it! This homemade trail mix is a delicious and nutritious snack that's perfect for hiking, packing in lunchboxes, or just enjoying as a healthy treat.

The combination of nuts, seeds, dried fruit, and chocolate provides a great balance of protein, healthy fats, fiber, and a touch of sweetness. You can easily customize the ingredients to your liking • try adding other dried fruits, roasted chickpeas, pretzels, or your favorite nuts and seeds.

This is a fun and easy recipe for young chefs to make. They'll enjoy mixing up the different ingredients and creating their own personalized trail mix blend.

64. Popcorn

Ingredient:

• 1/4 cup popcorn kernels
• 1•2 tbsp olive oil or coconut oil
• Salt (or other desired seasonings)

Equipment:
• Large pot with a lid
• Popcorn popper (optional)

Instructions:

1. If using a popcorn popper, follow the manufacturer's instructions. If using a pot, continue with the following steps.

2. In a large pot with a tight•fitting lid, heat the oil over medium•high heat.

3. Once the oil is hot, add the popcorn kernels in a single layer. Cover the pot with the lid.

4. Allow the kernels to pop, shaking the pot occasionally to prevent burning. Once the popping slows to 2•3 seconds between pops, remove the pot from the heat.

5. Carefully remove the lid, as hot steam will escape. Transfer the popped popcorn to a large bowl.

6. Season the popcorn with salt or any other desired seasonings, such as:
   • Garlic powder
   • Onion powder
   • Chili powder
   • Grated Parmesan cheese
   • Dried herbs (e.g., rosemary, thyme)

7. Toss the popcorn to evenly distribute the seasoning.

8. Serve the popcorn warm and enjoy!

Encourage the young chef to experiment with different seasoning combinations and to be careful when handling the hot pot. Popcorn is a great way to get kids involved in the kitchen and learn about the science of how popcorn pops!

65. Greek Yogurt with Honey

Ingredient:

• 1 cup plain Greek yogurt
• 2•3 tablespoons honey
• Fresh fruit (such as berries, sliced peaches, or diced mango), optional

Instructions:

1. Scoop the Greek yogurt into a bowl or individual serving dish.

2. Drizzle the honey over the top of the yogurt. Start with 2 tablespoons of honey and add more to taste, if desired.

3. If using fresh fruit, gently fold it into the yogurt and honey mixture.

4. Serve the Greek Yogurt with Honey immediately, or refrigerate until ready to enjoy.

That's it! This recipe is perfect for young chefs because it's:

• Simple to make with just 2•3 ingredients
• Customizable with different fruit toppings
• Healthy, with the protein•rich Greek yogurt and natural sweetness of honey
• Easy to adjust the honey amount to the child's taste preference

Encourage the young chef to experiment with different fruit combinations, such as strawberries and blueberries, or diced peaches and mango. They can also try adding a sprinkle of granola or chopped nuts for some extra crunch.

This Greek Yogurt with Honey is a delicious and nutritious snack or breakfast that's sure to be a hit with young chefs. Enjoy!

66. Cheese and Crackers

Ingredient:

• Assorted crackers (such as whole wheat, Triscuits, or Ritz)
• Sliced or cubed cheese (such as cheddar, Gouda, or Swiss)
• Optional toppings:
  • Grapes or apple slices
  • Olives
  • Nuts
  • Dried fruit

Instructions:

1. Arrange the assorted crackers on a serving plate or board.

2. Place the sliced or cubed cheese next to the crackers.

3. If using any optional toppings, arrange them around the crackers and cheese.

4. Encourage the young chef to assemble the cheese and crackers in a creative and visually appealing way.

That's it! This Cheese and Crackers snack is perfect for young chefs because:

• It's incredibly simple to prepare
• It allows for creativity in the presentation
• It's a healthy and satisfying snack
• It's easy to customize with different types of crackers, cheeses, and toppings

Encourage the young chef to experiment with different cheese and cracker combinations. They can try pairing sharp cheddar with whole wheat crackers, or creamy Brie with buttery Ritz crackers. Adding fresh fruit, olives, or nuts can also make the snack more interesting and nutritious.

This Cheese and Crackers recipe is a great way to get kids involved in the kitchen and teach them about building a balanced, tasty snack. Enjoy!

67. Fruit Salad

Ingredient:

- 1 cup diced pineapple
- 1 cup diced strawberries
- 1 cup diced mango
- 1 cup diced kiwi
- 1 cup blueberries
- 2 tbsp honey (optional)
- 1 tbsp fresh lemon juice

Instructions:

1. In a large bowl, combine the diced pineapple, strawberries, mango, kiwi, and blueberries.

2. If desired, drizzle the honey over the fruit and gently toss to coat.

3. Squeeze the lemon juice over the fruit salad and toss again to combine.

4. Cover the fruit salad and refrigerate for at least 30 minutes to allow the flavors to meld. Serve the chilled fruit salad in individual bowls or on a platter.

Tips for Young Chefs:

- Let the young chef help wash, peel, and dice the various fruits.
- Encourage them to be creative in arranging the colorful fruit in the bowl.
- Demonstrate how to safely use a knife to cut the softer fruits, like kiwi and strawberries.
- Have them measure and add the honey and lemon juice, tasting the salad to see if it needs more.

This Fruit Salad is a great recipe for young chefs because:

- It's easy to make with simple, fresh ingredients.
- It allows for creativity in choosing and arranging the different fruits.
- It's a healthy and delicious snack or dessert.
- The sweet and tangy flavors are sure to be a hit with kids.

Encourage the young chef to experiment with different fruit combinations, such as adding grapes, apple slices, or berries. They can also try drizzling a bit of yogurt or sprinkling some toasted nuts over the top.

68. Roasted Chickpeas

Ingredient:

• 1 (15 oz) can chickpeas (garbanzo beans), drained and rinsed
• 1 tbsp olive oil
• 1 tsp ground cumin
• 1 tsp paprika
• 1/2 tsp garlic powder
• 1/4 tsp salt

Instructions:

1. Preheat your oven to 400°F (200°C). Line a baking sheet with parchment paper.

2. Drain and rinse the chickpeas, then pat them dry with paper towels or a clean kitchen towel.

3. In a medium bowl, toss the chickpeas with the olive oil, cumin, paprika, garlic powder, and salt until they are evenly coated.

4. Spread the seasoned chickpeas in a single layer on the prepared baking sheet.

5. Roast the chickpeas in the preheated oven for 20•25 minutes, stirring halfway, until they are crispy and golden brown.

6. Remove the roasted chickpeas from the oven and let them cool for 5 minutes before serving.

Tips for Young Chefs:

• Let the young chef help measure and add the spices to the chickpeas.
• Encourage them to toss the chickpeas in the bowl to evenly coat them with the seasoning.
• Have them carefully spread the chickpeas out on the baking sheet.
• Remind them to be cautious when handling the hot baking sheet after it comes out of the oven.

Roasted Chickpeas are a great snack for young chefs because:

• They're easy to make with just a few simple ingredients.
• The kids can get hands•on experience with mixing and seasoning the chickpeas.
• The crunchy texture and flavorful spices make them a delicious and healthy snack.
• Chickpeas are a good source of protein, fiber, and other nutrients.

69. Granola Bars

Ingredient:

- 2 cups old•fashioned oats
- 1/2 cup chopped nuts (such as almonds, walnuts, or pecans)
- 1/2 cup shredded coconut (optional)
- 1/4 cup honey
- 1/4 cup brown sugar
- 1/4 cup peanut butter (or other nut butter)
- 1 tsp vanilla extract
- 1/4 tsp salt

Instructions:

1. Preheat your oven to 325°F (165°C). Line an 8x8 inch baking pan with parchment paper, leaving some overhang on the sides for easy removal.

2. In a large bowl, combine the oats, chopped nuts, and shredded coconut (if using). Stir to mix well.

3. In a small saucepan, heat the honey, brown sugar, peanut butter, and vanilla extract over medium heat, stirring constantly, until the mixture is smooth and well combined.

4. Pour the honey•peanut butter mixture over the oat mixture and stir until everything is evenly coated.

5. Transfer the granola mixture to the prepared baking pan and press it down firmly and evenly with a spatula or your hands.

6. Bake the granola bars in the preheated oven for 20•25 minutes, or until the edges are lightly golden brown.

7. Remove the pan from the oven and let the granola bars cool completely in the pan, about 1 hour.

8. Once cooled, use the parchment paper overhang to lift the granola bars out of the pan. Cut them into individual bars or squares.

9. Store the granola bars in an airtight container at room temperature for up to 1 week.

70. Guacamole with Tortilla Chips

Ingredient:

• 3 ripe avocados, pitted and diced
• 1/2 red onion, finely chopped
• 1 jalapeño, seeded and finely chopped (optional)
• 2 cloves garlic, minced
• 1/4 cup chopped fresh cilantro
• 2 tbsp fresh lime juice
• 1 tsp salt
• 1/4 tsp ground cumin

Tortilla Chips:
• 1 bag of your favorite tortilla chips

Instructions:
For the Guacamole:
1. In a medium bowl, gently mix together the diced avocados, chopped onion, jalapeño (if using), minced garlic, cilantro, lime juice, salt, and cumin.
2. Mash some of the avocado chunks with a fork or potato masher, leaving some larger pieces for texture.
3. Taste the guacamole and adjust seasoning as needed, adding more lime juice, salt, or cumin to your liking.

For the Tortilla Chips:
1. Open the bag of tortilla chips and arrange them on a serving platter or in a bowl.

To Serve:
1. Transfer the prepared guacamole to a serving bowl and place it next to the tortilla chips.
2. Encourage the young chef to scoop up the guacamole with the tortilla chips and enjoy!

This Guacamole with Tortilla Chips is a fun and easy recipe for young chefs to make. They'll enjoy mashing the avocados, mixing in the flavorful ingredients, and then dipping the crispy tortilla chips into the creamy guacamole.

You can also encourage the young chef to experiment with different mix•ins, such as diced tomatoes, corn, or black beans, to customize the guacamole to their taste. Enjoy this delicious and healthy snack!

71. Edamame

Ingredient:

• 1 lb fresh or frozen edamame in the pod
• 1•2 tsp coarse sea salt or kosher salt

Instructions:

1. If using frozen edamame, bring a large pot of water to a boil. Add the frozen edamame and cook for 3•5 minutes, until heated through and tender.

2. If using fresh edamame, bring a large pot of water to a boil. Add the fresh edamame pods and cook for 5•7 minutes, until tender.

3. Drain the cooked edamame in a colander and transfer to a serving bowl.

4. Sprinkle the cooked edamame with the coarse sea salt or kosher salt. Start with 1 teaspoon of salt and add more to taste.

5. Serve the salted edamame warm or at room temperature. Provide small bowls for the shells as the edamame is eaten.

Tips for Young Chefs:

• Let the young chef help measure and add the salt to the cooked edamame.
• Encourage them to taste the edamame and add more salt if desired.
• Explain that the edamame pods are not eaten, only the beans inside.
• Demonstrate how to pop the edamame beans out of the pods using their teeth or fingers.

Edamame is a great snack for young chefs because it's:

• Easy to prepare with just a few simple steps
• Nutritious, with protein, fiber, and vitamins
• Fun to eat, as the kids can pop the beans out of the pods
• Customizable with different seasonings (try garlic powder, lemon pepper, or chili powder)

Enjoy this healthy and delicious edamame snack!

72. Smoothie Popsicles

Ingredient:

• 1 cup frozen fruit (such as strawberries, blueberries, or mango)
• 1 cup milk (dairy, almond, or oat milk)
• 1/2 cup plain Greek yogurt
• 1•2 tbsp honey (optional)

Instructions:

1. In a blender, combine the frozen fruit, milk, and Greek yogurt. Blend until smooth and creamy.

2. Taste the smoothie and add honey if desired, blending again to incorporate.

3. Carefully pour the smoothie mixture into popsicle molds, leaving a small amount of space at the top for expansion.

4. Insert popsicle sticks into the molds, making sure they are centered.

5. Freeze the popsicles for at least 4 hours, or until completely frozen.

6. To remove the popsicles from the molds, run the molds under warm water for a few seconds, then gently pull the popsicles out.

Tips for Young Chefs:

• Let the young chef help choose the fruit and milk for the smoothie.
• Encourage them to taste the smoothie mixture and decide if they want to add honey.
• Have them carefully pour the smoothie into the popsicle molds.
• Let them insert the popsicle sticks and place the molds in the freezer.
• When the popsicles are ready, the young chef can help remove them from the molds.

These Smoothie Popsicles are a fun and healthy treat that kids will love to make and eat. The combination of fresh fruit, creamy yogurt, and sweet honey creates a delicious frozen treat. Enjoy!

73. Nut Butter Energy Balls

Ingredient:

• 1 cup rolled oats
• 1/2 cup nut butter (such as peanut, almond, or cashew butter)
• 1/4 cup honey
• 1/4 cup ground flaxseed (or chia seeds)
• 1/4 cup mini chocolate chips or chopped nuts (optional)

Instructions:

1. In a medium bowl, combine the rolled oats, nut butter, honey, and ground flaxseed (or chia seeds). Mix until well combined.

2. If using, stir in the mini chocolate chips or chopped nuts.

3. Using a small cookie scoop or your hands, form the mixture into small, bite•sized balls.

4. Place the energy balls on a parchment•lined baking sheet or plate.

5. Refrigerate the energy balls for at least 30 minutes to allow them to firm up.

6. Once chilled, the energy balls are ready to enjoy! Store them in an airtight container in the refrigerator for up to 1 week.

These Nut Butter Energy Balls are perfect for young chefs because:

• They're easy to make with just a few simple ingredients.
• The nut butter and oats provide a good source of protein and fiber.
• The honey adds natural sweetness.
• The optional mix•ins, like chocolate chips or nuts, allow for customization.
• They're a healthy, portable snack that kids will love.

Encourage the young chef to experiment with different nut butters and mix•ins to find their favorite combination. They can also get creative by rolling the energy balls in shredded coconut, cocoa powder, or crushed graham crackers.

These Nut Butter Energy Balls are a great way to get kids involved in the kitchen and teach them about making nutritious, homemade snacks.

74. Vegetable Chips

Ingredient:

• 2•3 medium vegetables (such as potatoes, sweet potatoes, zucchini, or beets)
• 1•2 tbsp olive oil or avocado oil
• Salt and other seasonings (such as garlic powder, paprika, or chili powder)

Instructions:

1. Preheat your oven to 375°F (190°C). Line 1•2 baking sheets with parchment paper.

2. Wash and peel the vegetables, if desired. Slice them into very thin, even slices using a sharp knife, a mandoline slicer, or a vegetable peeler.

3. Pat the vegetable slices dry with paper towels or a clean kitchen towel.

4. In a large bowl, toss the vegetable slices with the oil, making sure they are all lightly coated.

5. Arrange the oiled vegetable slices in a single layer on the prepared baking sheets, making sure they are not overlapping.

6. Sprinkle the vegetable slices with salt and any other desired seasonings.

7. Bake the vegetable chips in the preheated oven for 15•25 minutes, flipping them halfway, until they are crispy and lightly browned.

8. Keep a close eye on the chips towards the end of the baking time to prevent burning.

9. Remove the baked vegetable chips from the oven and let them cool completely before serving.

Tips for Young Chefs:

• Let the young chef help choose which vegetables to use and assist with the slicing.
• Have them toss the vegetable slices with the oil in the bowl.
• Encourage them to be creative with the seasoning blends.
• Remind them to be careful when handling the hot baking sheets.

75. Baked Sweet Potato Fries

Ingredient:

- 2 medium sweet potatoes, peeled and cut into 1/2•inch thick fry shapes
- 2 tbsp olive oil
- 1 tsp paprika
- 1/2 tsp garlic powder
- 1/2 tsp salt

Instructions:

1. Preheat your oven to 400°F (200°C). Line a baking sheet with parchment paper.

2. In a large bowl, toss the sweet potato fry shapes with the olive oil, paprika, garlic powder, and salt until they are evenly coated.

3. Spread the seasoned sweet potato fries in a single layer on the prepared baking sheet, making sure they are not overlapping.

4. Bake the sweet potato fries in the preheated oven for 20•25 minutes, flipping them halfway, until they are crispy and lightly browned.

5. Remove the baked sweet potato fries from the oven and let them cool for a few minutes before serving.

Tips for Young Chefs:

- Let the young chef help peel and cut the sweet potatoes into fry shapes.
- Have them toss the sweet potato fries with the oil and seasonings in the bowl.
- Encourage them to be careful when handling the hot baking sheet.
- Remind them to flip the fries halfway through the baking time.

Baked Sweet Potato Fries are a great recipe for young chefs because:

- It's a fun, hands•on activity to prepare.
- Sweet potatoes are a nutritious and delicious ingredient.
- The crispy, flavorful fries make a healthy and satisfying snack or side dish.
- The recipe is easy to follow and customize with different seasonings.

Enjoy these homemade Baked Sweet Potato Fries!

76. Cottage Cheese with Pineapple

Ingredient:

• 1 cup low•fat or non•fat cottage cheese
• 1/2 cup diced fresh pineapple (or canned pineapple tidbits, drained)
• Optional toppings:
  • Honey or maple syrup
  • Chopped nuts (such as almonds or walnuts)
  • Shredded coconut

Instructions:

1. In a small bowl, scoop the cottage cheese.

2. Top the cottage cheese with the diced pineapple.

3. If desired, drizzle a small amount of honey or maple syrup over the top.

4. Sprinkle any optional toppings, such as chopped nuts or shredded coconut, over the cottage cheese and pineapple.

That's it! This Cottage Cheese with Pineapple is a simple and nutritious snack that's perfect for young chefs.

Here's why it's great for kids:

• Cottage cheese is a good source of protein, calcium, and other nutrients.
• Pineapple adds natural sweetness and vitamin C.
• The optional toppings can add extra flavor, texture, and nutrients.
• It's easy to prepare and customize to individual tastes.

Encourage the young chef to experiment with different fruit combinations, such as diced mango, berries, or kiwi. They can also try adding a sprinkle of cinnamon or a drizzle of honey for extra flavor.

This Cottage Cheese with Pineapple is a healthy, delicious, and kid•friendly snack that's sure to be a hit.

77. Celery with Peanut Butter

Ingredient:

• 3•4 stalks of celery, washed and cut into 4•inch sticks
• 2•3 tablespoons of creamy peanut butter

Instructions:

1. Wash the celery stalks and pat them dry with a paper towel. Cut each stalk into 4•inch long sticks.

2. Spread about 1•2 teaspoons of peanut butter onto the end of each celery stick.

3. Arrange the peanut butter•filled celery sticks on a plate or in a container.

That's it! This snack is ready to enjoy.

Tips:
• Use natural, unsweetened peanut butter for a healthier option.

• For a fun twist, you can also try other nut or seed butters like almond butter or sunflower seed butter.

• Sprinkle a few raisins, dried cranberries, or mini chocolate chips on top of the peanut butter for extra flavor.

• Store any leftover celery sticks in the refrigerator for up to 3•4 days.

Celery with peanut butter is a classic, nutritious snack that provides a nice crunch and a boost of protein and healthy fats. It's a great option for kids and adults alike!

78. Almonds and Dried Fruit

Ingredient:

• 1 cup raw almonds
• 1/2 cup mixed dried fruit (such as raisins, apricots, cranberries, etc.)

Instructions:

1. In a small bowl, combine the raw almonds and dried fruit.

2. Stir to mix everything together.

That's it! This makes a great portable, nutrient•dense snack.

Some tips:

• Use a variety of dried fruits for different flavors and textures.

• You can also add a sprinkle of cinnamon or a pinch of sea salt for extra flavor.

• For a sweeter treat, you can drizzle a small amount of honey over the top.

• Store the mixture in an airtight container at room temperature for up to 1 week.

The combination of protein•rich almonds and naturally sweet dried fruit makes this a satisfying and healthy snack. It's perfect for packing in lunchboxes, taking on hikes, or keeping on hand for a quick energy boost.

79. Chocolate·Dipped Strawberries

Ingredient:

• 12•16 fresh strawberries, washed and patted dry
• 1 cup semisweet chocolate chips or chopped chocolate
• 1 tbsp coconut oil or vegetable shortening (optional, helps chocolate harden)

Instructions:

1. Line a baking sheet with parchment paper or a silicone baking mat.

2. In a small microwave•safe bowl, melt the chocolate chips and coconut oil (if using) in the microwave, stirring every 30 seconds, until smooth.

3. Holding them by the stem, dip each strawberry into the melted chocolate, coating about 3/4 of the berry.

4. Gently tap off any excess chocolate and place the dipped strawberries on the prepared baking sheet.

5. Refrigerate the strawberries for at least 30 minutes to allow the chocolate to harden.

6. Serve chilled. Store any leftovers in the refrigerator.

Tips:
• Let young chefs help dip the strawberries in the chocolate.
• Sprinkle with crushed nuts, sprinkles, or drizzle with white chocolate for extra decoration.
• Use milk, dark, or white chocolate depending on preference.

Enjoy these easy and delicious chocolate•dipped strawberries!

80. Mini Caprese Skewers

Ingredient:

• 12•16 cherry or grape tomatoes
• 12•16 small fresh mozzarella balls (bocconcini)
• 12•16 fresh basil leaves
• Balsamic glaze or reduction (optional)
• Toothpicks or small skewers

Instructions:

1. Wash and dry the tomatoes and basil leaves.

2. Thread the ingredients onto the toothpicks or skewers, alternating a tomato, a mozzarella ball, and a basil leaf.

3. Arrange the mini caprese skewers on a serving platter.

4. Drizzle a small amount of balsamic glaze or reduction over the top of the skewers, if desired.

That's it! The mini caprese skewers are ready to serve.

Tips:
• Use the smallest tomatoes and mozzarella balls you can find for the perfect bite•sized portions.

• For a more colorful presentation, use a variety of colored cherry tomatoes.

• Sprinkle a little salt and pepper over the skewers before serving.

• Serve the skewers chilled or at room temperature.

• This is a great make•ahead appetizer • assemble the skewers up to a day in advance and refrigerate until ready to serve.

The combination of juicy tomatoes, creamy mozzarella, and fresh basil makes these mini caprese skewers a delicious and visually appealing snack or appetizer. Enjoy!

81. Chocolate Chip Cookies

Ingredient:

• 2 1/4 cups all•purpose flour
• 1 teaspoon baking soda
• 1 teaspoon salt
• 1 cup unsalted butter, softened
• 3/4 cup granulated sugar
• 3/4 cup packed brown sugar
• 1 teaspoon vanilla extract
• 2 large eggs
• 2 cups semi•sweet chocolate chips

Instructions:

1. Preheat the oven to 375°F. Line baking sheets with parchment paper.

2. In a medium bowl, whisk together the flour, baking soda, and salt. Set aside.

3. In a large bowl, beat the butter and both sugars together until light and fluffy, about 2•3 minutes. Beat in the vanilla and then the eggs one at a time until combined.

4. Gradually stir the dry ingredients into the wet ingredients until just combined. Fold in the chocolate chips.

5. Scoop rounded tablespoons of dough onto the prepared baking sheets, spacing them about 2 inches apart.

6. Bake for 9•11 minutes, until the edges are set but the centers are still slightly soft.

7. Allow the cookies to cool on the baking sheets for 5 minutes before transferring to a wire rack to cool completely.

Tips:
• For chewier cookies, use more brown sugar. For crispier cookies, use more granulated sugar.
• Chill the dough for 30 minutes before baking for thicker, chewier cookies.
• Try different mix•ins like nuts, M&Ms, or chopped candy bars.
• Store cookies in an airtight container for up to 1 week.

Enjoy these classic, homemade chocolate chip cookies!

82. Brownies

Ingredient:

• 1/2 cup (1 stick) unsalted butter, melted
• 1 cup granulated sugar
• 2 large eggs
• 1 tsp vanilla extract
• 1/3 cup all•purpose flour
• 1/4 cup unsweetened cocoa powder
• 1/4 tsp salt
• 1/2 cup semi•sweet chocolate chips (optional)

Instructions:

1. Preheat your oven to 350°F (175°C). Grease an 8x8 inch baking pan with butter or non•stick cooking spray.

2. In a medium bowl, whisk together the melted butter and granulated sugar until combined.

3. Add the eggs one at a time, whisking well after each addition. Then stir in the vanilla extract.

4. In a separate bowl, whisk together the flour, cocoa powder, and salt.

5. Gradually add the dry ingredients to the wet ingredients, mixing just until combined. Do not overmix.

6. If using, fold in the chocolate chips.

7. Spread the brownie batter evenly into the prepared baking pan.

8. Bake the brownies in the preheated oven for 20•25 minutes, or until a toothpick inserted in the center comes out with a few moist crumbs. Allow the brownies to cool completely in the pan before cutting and serving.

Tips for Young Chefs:

• Let the young chef help measure and mix the ingredients.
• Demonstrate how to properly whisk the wet and dry ingredients.
• Encourage them to be gentle when folding in the chocolate chips.
• Remind them to be careful when handling the hot baking pan.

83. Fruit Tart

Ingredient:

- 1 1/4 cups all•purpose flour
- 1/2 cup unsalted butter, chilled and cubed
- 1/4 cup granulated sugar
- 1 egg yolk
- 1•2 tbsp cold water

Filling Ingredients:

- 8 oz cream cheese, softened
- 1/2 cup powdered sugar
- 1 tsp vanilla extract
- Assorted fresh fruit (such as strawberries, kiwi, blueberries, mandarin oranges)
- Apricot glaze (optional)

Instructions:

Crust:

1. In a food processor, pulse the flour, butter, and sugar until mixture resembles coarse crumbs.
2. Add the egg yolk and 1 tbsp of water, pulsing until the dough just begins to hold together. Add more water as needed.
3. Shape the dough into a disk, wrap in plastic, and refrigerate for at least 30 minutes.
4. Roll out the dough and press into a 9•inch tart pan with a removable bottom. Prick the bottom with a fork.
5. Bake at 375ºF for 12•15 minutes until lightly golden. Allow to cool completely.

Filling:

1. In a medium bowl, beat the cream cheese, powdered sugar, and vanilla until smooth and creamy.
2. Spread the cream cheese mixture evenly into the cooled tart shell.

Assembly:

1. Arrange the assorted fresh fruit in a decorative pattern on top of the cream cheese filling.
2. If desired, heat some apricot preserves with a splash of water until warm and glossy. Brush the fruit with the glaze.
3. Refrigerate the tart for at least 2 hours before serving.

Tips:

- Use a variety of colorful, seasonal fruits for the best presentation.
- The tart can be made a day in advance and refrigerated until ready to serve.
- Serve chilled or at room temperature.

84. Apple Pie

Ingredient:

• 2 1/2 cups all•purpose flour
• 1 tsp salt
• 2/3 cup chilled unsalted butter, cubed
• 1/4 cup ice water

Filling Ingredients:
• 6•8 Granny Smith or other tart apples, peeled, cored and sliced
• 3/4 cup granulated sugar
• 2 tbsp all•purpose flour
• 1 tsp ground cinnamon
• 1/4 tsp ground nutmeg
• 1 tbsp unsalted butter, cubed

Instructions:
Crust:
1. In a food processor, pulse the flour and salt. Add the butter and pulse until mixture resembles coarse meal.
2. Add the ice water 1 tbsp at a time, pulsing just until the dough begins to hold together.
3. Divide the dough in half, shape each into a disk, wrap in plastic and refrigerate for at least 1 hour.

Filling: In a large bowl, toss the apple slices with the sugar, flour, cinnamon and nutmeg until well coated.

Assembly:
1. On a lightly floured surface, roll out one disk of dough into a 12•inch circle. Fit into a 9•inch pie plate.
2. Spoon the apple filling into the crust and dot the top with the cubed butter.
3. Roll out the remaining dough into a 12•inch circle for the top crust. Place over the filling and crimp the edges to seal.
4. Cut slits in the top crust to allow steam to escape.
5. Bake at 425ºF for 25 minutes. Reduce heat to 350ºF and bake for 30•40 minutes more, until the crust is golden brown.
6. Allow to cool completely before slicing and serving.

Tips:
• For a flakier crust, use a combination of butter and shortening.
• Brush the top crust with an egg wash for a shiny finish.
• Serve with vanilla ice cream or whipped cream.

85. Vanilla Cupcakes

Ingredient:

- 1 1/2 cups all•purpose flour
- 1 tsp baking powder
- 1/4 tsp salt
- 1/2 cup (1 stick) unsalted butter, softened
- 3/4 cup granulated sugar
- 2 large eggs
- 1 tsp vanilla extract
- 1/2 cup milk

Frosting:

- 1/2 cup (1 stick) unsalted butter, softened
- 3 cups powdered sugar
- 2 tbsp milk
- 1 tsp vanilla extract

Instructions:
For the Cupcakes:

1. Preheat your oven to 350°F (175°C). Line a 12•cup muffin tin with paper liners.

2. In a medium bowl, whisk together the flour, baking powder, and salt. Set aside.

3. In a large bowl, use a hand mixer to cream the butter and sugar together until light and fluffy, about 2•3 minutes.

4. Beat in the eggs one at a time, then stir in the vanilla extract.

5. Alternate adding the flour mixture and milk to the butter mixture, mixing just until combined after each addition.

6. Divide the batter evenly among the prepared muffin cups, filling them about 3/4 full.

7. Bake the cupcakes for 18•20 minutes, or until a toothpick inserted in the center comes out clean.

8. Allow the cupcakes to cool in the tin for 5 minutes, then transfer them to a wire rack to cool completely.

For the Frosting:
1. In a large bowl, use a hand mixer to beat the butter until smooth and creamy.
2. Gradually add the powdered sugar, 1 cup at a time, beating well after each addition.
3. Mix in the milk and vanilla extract until the frosting is light and fluffy.

To Assemble:
1. Once the cupcakes are completely cooled, use a piping bag or a knife to frost the tops of the cupcakes.
2. Decorate the frosted cupcakes with sprinkles, if desired.

86. Banana Bread

Ingredient:

- 1 3/4 cups all•purpose flour
- 1 teaspoon baking soda
- 1/4 teaspoon salt
- 1/2 cup unsalted butter, softened
- 3/4 cup granulated sugar
- 2 large eggs
- 1 teaspoon vanilla extract
- 1 1/4 cups mashed ripe bananas (about 3 medium)

Instructions:

1. Preheat the oven to 350°F. Grease a 9x5•inch loaf pan.

2. In a medium bowl, whisk together the flour, baking soda, and salt. Set aside.

3. In a large bowl, beat the butter and sugar together until light and fluffy, about 2•3 minutes. Beat in the eggs one at a time, then stir in the vanilla and mashed bananas.

4. Gradually fold the dry ingredients into the wet ingredients just until combined, being careful not to overmix.

5. Pour the batter into the prepared loaf pan and smooth the top.

6. Bake for 55•65 minutes, until a toothpick inserted in the center comes out clean.

7. Allow the banana bread to cool in the pan for 10 minutes, then transfer to a wire rack to cool completely before slicing.

Tips:
- For extra moisture, add 1/4 cup sour cream or yogurt to the batter.
- Fold in chopped walnuts, pecans, or chocolate chips for extra flavor.
- Sprinkle the top with a little cinnamon or nutmeg before baking.
- Wrap tightly and store at room temperature for up to 4 days.

This classic banana bread is moist, flavorful, and perfect for breakfast, snacking, or dessert. Enjoy!

87. Cheesecake

Ingredient:

• 1 1/2 cups graham cracker crumbs
• 5 tbsp unsalted butter, melted

Filling Ingredients:
• 24 oz (3 packages) cream cheese, softened
• 1 cup granulated sugar
• 1/4 cup sour cream
• 1 tsp vanilla extract
• 2 large eggs

Instructions:

For the Crust:
1. Preheat your oven to 325°F (165°C). Grease a 9·inch springform pan.
2. In a medium bowl, mix together the graham cracker crumbs and melted butter until well combined.
3. Press the crumb mixture firmly into the bottom and slightly up the sides of the prepared springform pan.

For the Filling:
1. In a large bowl, use a hand mixer or stand mixer to beat the cream cheese until light and fluffy, about 2·3 minutes.
2. Gradually add the sugar and beat until smooth, scraping down the sides as needed.
3. Mix in the sour cream and vanilla extract until combined.
4. Add the eggs one at a time, beating well after each addition.

Baking:
1. Pour the cheesecake filling into the prepared graham cracker crust.
2. Bake the cheesecake in the preheated oven for 55·65 minutes, or until the center is almost set.
3. Turn off the oven and leave the cheesecake inside with the door closed for 1 hour.
4. Remove the cheesecake from the oven and allow it to cool completely on a wire rack, then refrigerate for at least 4 hours or overnight before serving.

Tips for Young Chefs:
• Let the young chef help measure and mix the crust ingredients.
• Demonstrate how to press the crust into the springform pan.
• Have them assist with mixing the filling ingredients.
• Remind them to be gentle when pouring the filling into the crust.
• Explain the importance of the slow cooling process for the perfect cheesecake texture

88. Pumpkin Pie

Ingredient:

• 1 (15 oz) can pumpkin puree
• 1 (14 oz) can sweetened condensed milk
• 2 large eggs
• 1 tsp ground cinnamon
• 1/2 tsp ground ginger
• 1/4 tsp ground nutmeg
• 1/4 tsp salt
• 1 (9•inch) unbaked pie crust

Instructions:

1. Preheat the oven to 425ºF.

2. In a large bowl, whisk together the pumpkin puree, sweetened condensed milk, eggs, cinnamon, ginger, nutmeg, and salt until well combined.

3. Pour the pumpkin filling into the unbaked pie crust.

4. Bake for 15 minutes at 425ºF. Then reduce the oven temperature to 350ºF and bake for 40•45 minutes more, until the center is almost set.

5. Allow the pie to cool completely, at least 2 hours, before slicing and serving.

Tips for Young Chefs:
• Let the kids help measure and mix the ingredients.
• Have them carefully pour the filling into the pie crust.
• Supervise them when putting the pie in and taking it out of the oven.
• Discuss food safety, like not eating raw eggs.
• Encourage them to get creative with toppings like whipped cream, caramel sauce, or a sprinkle of cinnamon.

This classic pumpkin pie is easy to make and a great baking project for young chefs. The simple ingredients and step•by•step instructions make it a fun and rewarding recipe to try.

89. Chocolate Mousse

Ingredient:

• 4 oz semisweet chocolate, chopped
• 2 large egg whites
• 2 tbsp granulated sugar
• 1 cup heavy cream

Instructions:

1. In a medium heatproof bowl, melt the chopped chocolate over a pot of simmering water, stirring occasionally until smooth. Remove from heat and let cool slightly.

2. In a medium bowl, beat the egg whites with an electric mixer until foamy. Gradually add the sugar and continue beating until stiff peaks form.

3. In a separate bowl, beat the heavy cream with an electric mixer until stiff peaks form.

4. Gently fold the whipped cream into the melted chocolate until just combined. Then gently fold in the whipped egg whites.

5. Spoon the chocolate mousse into individual serving dishes or glasses. Refrigerate for at least 2 hours before serving.

Tips for Young Chefs:
• Let the kids help measure and chop the chocolate.

• Have them take turns beating the egg whites and cream with the electric mixer (with supervision).

• Demonstrate how to gently fold the ingredients together.

• Encourage them to get creative with toppings like whipped cream, chocolate shavings, or fresh berries.

• Discuss food safety, like not eating raw eggs.

This light and airy chocolate mousse is a fun, easy, and delicious dessert for young chefs to make. The simple ingredients and hands•on steps make it a great baking project.

90. Lemon Bars

Ingredient:

• 1 cup all•purpose flour
• 1/2 cup unsalted butter, softened
• 1/4 cup powdered sugar

Filling Ingredients:
• 4 large eggs
• 1 1/4 cups granulated sugar
• 1/4 cup all•purpose flour
• 1/4 cup fresh lemon juice (about 2•3 lemons)
• 1 tbsp grated lemon zest
• 1/4 tsp salt

Instructions:
1. Preheat the oven to 350°F. Grease an 8x8•inch baking pan.

Crust:
2. In a medium bowl, use your fingers to mix together the flour, butter, and powdered sugar until it forms a crumbly dough.
3. Press the dough evenly into the bottom of the prepared baking pan.
4. Bake for 15•18 minutes, until lightly golden.

Filling:
5. In a medium bowl, whisk together the eggs, granulated sugar, flour, lemon juice, lemon zest, and salt until well combined.
6. Pour the lemon filling over the hot crust.
7. Bake for 20•25 minutes, until the center is set.

8. Allow the lemon bars to cool completely in the pan, then cut into squares.
9. Dust the tops with powdered sugar before serving.

Tips for Young Chefs:
• Let the kids help measure and mix the crust ingredients.
• Have them press the crust into the pan.
• Demonstrate how to zest and juice the lemons.
• Supervise them when whisking the filling ingredients.
• Encourage them to get creative with the powdered sugar topping.

These classic lemon bars are a great baking project for young chefs. The simple ingredients and steps make them easy to prepare, and the bright, tangy flavor is sure to be a hit!

91. Panna Cotta

Ingredient:

- 2 cups heavy cream
- 1 cup whole milk
- 1/2 cup granulated sugar
- 1 vanilla bean, split lengthwise (or 1 tsp vanilla extract)
- 2 1/4 tsp unflavored gelatin powder

For Serving (optional):
- Fresh berries
- Caramel sauce
- Chocolate shavings

Instructions:

1. In a medium saucepan, combine the heavy cream, milk, sugar, and vanilla bean. Heat over medium, stirring occasionally, until the sugar has dissolved and the mixture is steaming, about 5 minutes. Remove from heat and let the vanilla bean steep for 30 minutes.

2. Sprinkle the gelatin over 2 tablespoons of cold water in a small bowl. Let stand for 5 minutes to soften.

3. Remove the vanilla bean from the cream mixture. Whisk the softened gelatin into the warm cream until fully dissolved.

4. Lightly grease 6 ramekins or small bowls. Divide the panna cotta mixture evenly among them. Refrigerate for at least 4 hours, or until set.

5. To unmold, run a knife around the edge of each ramekin and invert onto a plate. Top with fresh berries, caramel sauce, chocolate shavings, or other desired toppings.

Tips:
- For a creamier texture, use all heavy cream instead of a milk/cream mixture.
- Substitute the vanilla bean with 1 tsp vanilla extract if desired.
- Garnish with fresh fruit, nuts, citrus zest, or a drizzle of honey.
- Panna cotta can be made 2•3 days in advance and refrigerated until ready to serve.

Enjoy this silky, elegant Italian dessert! The smooth, creamy panna cotta pairs beautifully with sweet and tangy toppings.

92. Peach Cobbler

Ingredient:

• 6 cups sliced fresh peaches (about 6•8 medium peaches)
• 1/2 cup granulated sugar
• 2 tbsp all•purpose flour
• 1 tsp ground cinnamon
• 1/4 tsp ground nutmeg

Topping Ingredients:
• 1 cup all•purpose flour
• 1/4 cup granulated sugar
• 2 tsp baking powder
• 1/4 tsp salt
• 6 tbsp cold unsalted butter, cubed
• 1/2 cup milk

Instructions:

1. Preheat the oven to 375ºF. Grease a 9x13•inch baking dish.

Filling:
2. In a large bowl, gently toss the sliced peaches with the sugar, flour, cinnamon, and nutmeg until well coated. Pour the filling into the prepared baking dish.

Topping:
3. In a medium bowl, whisk together the flour, sugar, baking powder, and salt.
4. Cut in the cold butter using a pastry blender or two forks until the mixture resembles coarse crumbs.
5. Stir in the milk just until a thick batter forms.
6. Dollop the batter over the peach filling, spreading it out gently.

7. Bake for 30•35 minutes, until the topping is golden brown and the filling is bubbly. Allow to cool for 15 minutes before serving. Serve warm, with vanilla ice cream if desired.

Tips for Young Chefs:
• Let the kids help wash, peel, and slice the peaches.
• Have them measure and mix the filling ingredients.
• Demonstrate how to cut in the cold butter for the topping.
• Supervise when adding the milk and spreading the topping.
• Encourage them to get creative with the presentation, like adding a scoop of ice cream

93. Raspberry Sorbet

Ingredient:

- 12 oz fresh or frozen raspberries
- 3/4 cup granulated sugar
- 1/4 cup water
- 1 tbsp lemon juice

Instructions:

1. In a medium saucepan, combine the sugar and water. Bring to a simmer over medium heat, stirring occasionally, until the sugar has fully dissolved. Remove from heat and let cool completely.

2. In a food processor or blender, puree the raspberries until smooth. Press the puree through a fine mesh strainer to remove the seeds.

3. In a medium bowl, whisk together the raspberry puree, cooled sugar syrup, and lemon juice until well combined.

4. Pour the raspberry mixture into an ice cream maker and churn according to manufacturer's instructions, usually 20•30 minutes, until thickened and frozen.

5. Transfer the sorbet to an airtight container and freeze for at least 2 hours before serving.

Tips:
- For a creamier texture, substitute 1/4 cup of the water with heavy cream or half•and•half.
- Add a splash of vodka or raspberry liqueur for an adult version.
- Garnish with fresh raspberries, mint leaves, or a drizzle of honey.
- Freeze the sorbet for up to 2 months.

This bright, refreshing raspberry sorbet is the perfect palate cleanser or light dessert on a warm day. Enjoy the sweet•tart flavor of fresh raspberries in this easy homemade treat!

94. Creme Brulee

Ingredient:

• 2 cups heavy cream
• 1 vanilla bean, split lengthwise (or 1 tsp vanilla extract)
• 5 large egg yolks
• 1/2 cup granulated sugar, plus more for caramelizing

Instructions:

1. Preheat the oven to 325ºF. Place four 6•oz ramekins in a baking dish.

2. In a medium saucepan, heat the heavy cream and vanilla bean (or extract) over medium heat, stirring occasionally, until steaming and bubbles start to form around the edge. Remove from heat and let sit for 30 minutes to infuse the vanilla flavor.

3. In a medium bowl, whisk the egg yolks and 1/2 cup sugar together until smooth and pale yellow.

4. Slowly pour the warm cream into the egg yolk mixture, whisking constantly.

5. Strain the custard through a fine mesh sieve to remove any cooked egg bits.

6. Carefully pour the custard into the ramekins, dividing it evenly.

7. Pour enough hot water into the baking dish to come halfway up the sides of the ramekins.

8. Bake for 30•35 minutes, until the centers are just set. The centers should still be slightly jiggly.

9. Remove the ramekins from the water bath and let cool completely, then refrigerate for at least 2 hours.

10. Just before serving, sprinkle an even layer of granulated sugar over the top of each chilled custard. Use a kitchen torch to caramelize the sugar until golden brown.

This classic crème brûlée is a fun and impressive dessert for young chefs to make with some adult assistance. The creamy custard and crisp caramelized sugar topping make it a delicious treat.

95. Chocolate Fondue

Ingredient:

- 12 oz semisweet chocolate, chopped
- 1 cup heavy cream
- 2 tbsp granulated sugar
- 1 tsp vanilla extract
- Pinch of salt

Dipping Suggestions:
- Strawberries
- Banana slices
- Marshmallows
- Pound cake cubes
- Pretzel rods
- Graham cracker sticks

Instructions:

1. In a medium heatproof bowl, combine the chopped chocolate, heavy cream, sugar, vanilla, and salt.

2. Set the bowl over a saucepan of simmering water, making sure the bottom of the bowl doesn't touch the water.

3. Stir the mixture constantly with a whisk or wooden spoon until the chocolate is completely melted and the fondue is smooth and creamy, about 5•7 minutes.

4. Remove the bowl from the saucepan and wipe any water droplets from the bottom of the bowl.

5. Transfer the warm chocolate fondue to a fondue pot or serving bowl. Keep it warm over a low flame or tea light.

6. Arrange the desired dipping items on a platter around the fondue pot.

7. Encourage everyone to dip the items into the warm chocolate fondue and enjoy!

Chocolate fondue is a fun, interactive dessert that kids will love making and eating. The simple ingredients and hands•on assembly make it a great recipe for young chefs.

96. Berry Parfait

Ingredient:

• 2 cups plain Greek yogurt
• 1/4 cup honey (or maple syrup)
• 1 tsp vanilla extract
• 2 cups mixed fresh berries (such as strawberries, blueberries, raspberries)
• 1/2 cup granola or toasted nuts

Instructions:

1. In a medium bowl, mix together the Greek yogurt, honey, and vanilla extract until well combined.

2. In parfait glasses or small bowls, layer the yogurt mixture, fresh berries, and granola or nuts, repeating the layers until you reach the top.

3. Refrigerate the parfaits for at least 30 minutes before serving to allow the flavors to meld.

4. Serve chilled.

Tips:
• Use a variety of fresh, seasonal berries for the best flavor and color.
• Substitute low•fat or non•fat Greek yogurt to make it lighter.
• For a creamier texture, use vanilla•flavored Greek yogurt.
• Sprinkle a little cinnamon or lemon zest over the top.
• Make these parfaits ahead of time and refrigerate until ready to serve.

The combination of creamy yogurt, sweet berries, and crunchy granola or nuts makes this berry parfait a delicious and nutritious breakfast, snack, or dessert. Enjoy!

97. Ice Cream Sandwiches

Ingredient:

• 1 cup all•purpose flour
• 1/2 cup unsweetened cocoa powder
• 1/2 tsp baking soda
• 1/4 tsp salt
• 1/2 cup unsalted butter, softened
• 3/4 cup granulated sugar
• 1 egg
• 1 tsp vanilla extract
• 1 pint vanilla ice cream

Instructions:

1. Preheat the oven to 350°F. Line two baking sheets with parchment paper.

2. In a medium bowl, whisk together the flour, cocoa powder, baking soda, and salt.

3. In a large bowl, beat the butter and sugar together until light and fluffy, about 2•3 minutes. Beat in the egg and vanilla.

4. Gradually stir the dry ingredients into the wet ingredients until just combined.

5. Scoop rounded tablespoons of dough onto the prepared baking sheets, spacing them about 2 inches apart.

6. Bake for 8•10 minutes, until the cookies are set. Allow to cool completely on the baking sheets.

7. Once cooled, place a small scoop of ice cream between two cookies to make a sandwich.

8. Wrap each ice cream sandwich individually in plastic wrap or foil and freeze for at least 2 hours before serving.

Tips for Young Chefs:
• Let the kids help measure and mix the cookie dough ingredients.
• Have them use a spoon or cookie scoop to portion the dough.
• Supervise when putting the cookies in and taking them out of the oven.
• Demonstrate how to assemble the ice cream sandwiches.
• Encourage creativity with different ice cream flavors or cookie varieties.

98. Oatmeal Raisin Cookies

Ingredient:

- 1 cup (2 sticks) unsalted butter, softened
- 1 cup packed brown sugar
- 1 egg
- 1 tsp vanilla extract
- 1 1/2 cups all•purpose flour
- 1 tsp baking soda
- 1/2 tsp ground cinnamon
- 1/4 tsp salt
- 3 cups old•fashioned oats
- 1 cup raisins

Instructions:

1. Preheat the oven to 350°F. Line two baking sheets with parchment paper.

2. In a large bowl, beat the butter and brown sugar together until light and fluffy, about 2•3 minutes. Beat in the egg and vanilla.

3. In a separate bowl, whisk together the flour, baking soda, cinnamon, and salt.

4. Gradually stir the dry ingredients into the wet ingredients until just combined. Fold in the oats and raisins.

5. Scoop rounded tablespoons of dough onto the prepared baking sheets, spacing them about 2 inches apart.

6. Bake for 10•12 minutes, until the edges are lightly golden.

7. Allow the cookies to cool on the baking sheets for 5 minutes before transferring to a wire rack to cool completely.

Tips for Young Chefs:
- Let the kids help measure and mix the ingredients.
- Have them use a spoon or cookie scoop to portion the dough.
- Supervise when putting the cookies in and taking them out of the oven.
- Encourage creativity with mix•ins like chocolate chips or chopped nuts.

These classic oatmeal raisin cookies are a delicious and easy recipe for young chefs to make. The simple steps and hands•on preparation make it a fun baking project.

99. Chocolate Cake

Ingredient:

• 2 cups all•purpose flour
• 2 cups granulated sugar
• 3/4 cup unsweetened cocoa powder
• 1 1/2 tsp baking powder
• 1 1/2 tsp baking soda
• 1 tsp salt
• 2 large eggs
• 1 cup milk
• 1/2 cup vegetable oil
• 2 tsp vanilla extract
• 1 cup boiling water

Frosting Ingredients:
• 1 cup unsalted butter, softened
• 3 cups powdered sugar
• 1/3 cup unsweetened cocoa powder
• 1/4 cup milk
• 1 tsp vanilla extract
• Pinch of salt

Instructions:

Cake:
1. Preheat the oven to 350°F. Grease and flour two 9•inch round cake pans.
2. In a large bowl, whisk together the flour, sugar, cocoa powder, baking powder, baking soda, and salt.
3. In a separate bowl, beat the eggs, milk, oil, and vanilla until combined.
4. Slowly add the wet ingredients to the dry ingredients and mix until just combined. Carefully stir in the boiling water.
5. Divide the batter evenly between the prepared cake pans.
6. Bake for 30•35 minutes, until a toothpick inserted in the center comes out clean.
7. Allow the cakes to cool in the pans for 10 minutes, then transfer to a wire rack to cool completely.

Frosting:
8. In a large bowl, beat the butter until light and fluffy. Gradually add the powdered sugar and cocoa powder, alternating with the milk, until smooth and creamy. Stir in the vanilla and salt.

Assembly:
9. Place one cake layer on a serving plate or cake stand. Spread half of the frosting evenly over the top.
10. Top with the second cake layer and spread the remaining frosting over the top and sides of the cake.

This classic chocolate cake is a delicious and fun baking project for young chefs. The simple steps and hands•on preparation make it a great way to get kids involved in the kitchen.

100. Strawberry Shortcake

Ingredient:

• 2 cups all•purpose flour
• 2 tablespoons granulated sugar
• 2 teaspoons baking powder
• 1/4 teaspoon salt
• 6 tablespoons cold unsalted butter, cubed
• 3/4 cup cold milk

Filling Ingredients:
• 1 lb fresh strawberries, hulled and sliced
• 2 tablespoons granulated sugar
• Whipped cream, for serving

Instructions:
Shortcake:
1. Preheat the oven to 400°F. Line a baking sheet with parchment paper.
2. In a large bowl, whisk together the flour, sugar, baking powder, and salt.
3. Cut in the cold butter using a pastry blender or two forks until mixture resembles coarse crumbs.
4. Stir in the cold milk just until a shaggy dough forms.
5. Turn the dough out onto a lightly floured surface and gently knead 2•3 times.
6. Pat the dough into a 6•inch round about 3/4•inch thick. Cut into 6 wedges and place on the prepared baking sheet.
7. Bake for 12•15 minutes, until golden brown. Allow to cool slightly.

Filling:
8. In a medium bowl, gently toss the sliced strawberries with the sugar. Let sit for 10 minutes to release juices.

Assembly:
9. Split each shortcake in half horizontally. Top the bottom halves with the sugared strawberries and their juices.
10. Add a dollop of whipped cream and replace the top halves.
11. Serve the strawberry shortcakes immediately.

This classic strawberry shortcake is a delicious and fun dessert for young chefs to make. The simple biscuit•like shortcakes and fresh strawberry filling make it a crowd•pleasing treat.

101. Coconut Macaroons

Ingredient:

- 3 large egg whites
- 1/2 cup granulated sugar
- 1/4 tsp salt
- 1 tsp vanilla extract
- 2 1/2 cups sweetened shredded coconut

Instructions:

1. Preheat the oven to 325°F. Line a baking sheet with parchment paper.

2. In a medium bowl, beat the egg whites with an electric mixer until they start to foam. Gradually add the sugar and salt, beating until stiff peaks form.

3. Gently fold in the vanilla and coconut until well combined.

4. Scoop rounded tablespoons of the coconut mixture and place them about 1 inch apart on the prepared baking sheet.

5. Bake for 18•20 minutes, until the macaroons are lightly golden on the edges.

6. Allow the macaroons to cool on the baking sheet for 5 minutes before transferring to a wire rack to cool completely.

Tips for Young Chefs:
- Let the kids help measure and mix the ingredients.

- Have them take turns beating the egg whites with the electric mixer (with supervision).

- Demonstrate how to gently fold in the coconut.

- Supervise when scooping and placing the macaroons on the baking sheet.

- Encourage creativity with decorations like drizzled chocolate or sprinkled coconut.

These classic coconut macaroons are a simple and delicious treat that young chefs will enjoy making. The easy steps and hands•on preparation make it a great baking project for kids.

102. Key Lime Pie

Ingredient:

• 1 1/2 cups graham cracker crumbs
• 5 tbsp unsalted butter, melted

Filling Ingredients:
• 1 (14 oz) can sweetened condensed milk
• 3 large egg yolks
• 1/2 cup fresh key lime juice (about 20•25 key limes)

Instructions:
Crust:
1. Preheat the oven to 350°F. Grease a 9•inch pie plate.
2. In a medium bowl, mix together the graham cracker crumbs and melted butter until well combined.
3. Press the crumb mixture evenly into the bottom and up the sides of the prepared pie plate.
4. Bake for 8•10 minutes, then let cool completely.

Filling:
5. In a medium bowl, whisk together the sweetened condensed milk and egg yolks until smooth.
6. Gradually whisk in the key lime juice until fully incorporated.
7. Pour the filling into the cooled graham cracker crust.

8. Bake for 15•18 minutes, until the center is set but still slightly jiggly.
9. Allow the pie to cool completely at room temperature, then refrigerate for at least 2 hours before serving.

Tips for Young Chefs:
• Let the kids help measure and mix the graham cracker crust ingredients.
• Demonstrate how to press the crust into the pie plate.
• Have them help squeeze the key limes and measure the juice.
• Supervise when whisking the filling ingredients and baking the pie.
• Encourage creativity with toppings like whipped cream or lime zest.

This classic key lime pie is a refreshing and easy dessert that young chefs will enjoy making. The simple steps and hands•on preparation make it a great baking project.

103. Bread Pudding

Ingredient:

- 8 cups cubed day•old bread (such as challah or brioche)
- 4 large eggs
- 2 cups whole milk
- 1 cup heavy cream
- 3/4 cup granulated sugar
- 1 tsp vanilla extract
- 1/2 tsp ground cinnamon
- 1/4 tsp ground nutmeg
- 1/4 tsp salt
- 1/2 cup raisins or chopped dried fruit (optional)

Sauce Ingredients:
- 1/2 cup unsalted butter
- 1/2 cup brown sugar
- 1/2 cup heavy cream
- 1 tsp vanilla extract

Instructions:

1. Preheat the oven to 350°F. Grease a 9x13•inch baking dish.

2. In a large bowl, whisk together the eggs, milk, cream, sugar, vanilla, cinnamon, nutmeg, and salt until well combined.

3. Gently fold in the cubed bread and raisins (if using) until the bread is evenly coated.

4. Transfer the bread pudding mixture to the prepared baking dish and spread it out evenly.

5. Bake for 45•55 minutes, until the center is set and the top is golden brown.

Sauce:
6. In a small saucepan, melt the butter over medium heat. Whisk in the brown sugar and cream. Bring to a simmer and cook for 2•3 minutes, stirring constantly, until thickened slightly.

7. Remove from heat and stir in the vanilla. Serve the warm bread pudding drizzled with the warm butter sauce.

104. Tiramisu

Ingredient:
- 4 large egg yolks
- 1/2 cup granulated sugar
- 1 lb mascarpone cheese
- 1 cup strong brewed coffee, cooled
- 2 tbsp coffee liqueur (such as Kahlua)
- 24•30 ladyfinger cookies
- Unsweetened cocoa powder, for dusting

Instructions:
1. In a medium heatproof bowl, whisk together the egg yolks and sugar until smooth.

2. Place the bowl over a saucepan of simmering water, making sure the bottom of the bowl doesn't touch the water. Whisk the mixture constantly until it thickens and reaches 160°F on a candy thermometer, about 5•7 minutes.

3. Remove the bowl from the heat and let the mixture cool completely, about 30 minutes.

4. In a large bowl, beat the mascarpone cheese with a hand mixer until smooth and creamy.

5. Gently fold the cooled egg yolk mixture into the mascarpone until well combined.

6. In a shallow bowl, combine the coffee and coffee liqueur.

7. One at a time, quickly dip the ladyfinger cookies into the coffee mixture, coating both sides. Arrange the soaked cookies in a single layer in an 8x8•inch baking dish.

8. Spread half of the mascarpone mixture over the ladyfingers. Dust with a thin layer of cocoa powder.

9. Repeat the layers of soaked ladyfingers and mascarpone, ending with a dusting of cocoa powder.

10. Cover and refrigerate the tiramisu for at least 6 hours, or up to 24 hours, before serving.

Tiramisu is a classic Italian dessert that young chefs can make with some adult assistance. The creamy mascarpone and coffee•soaked ladyfingers make it a delicious and impressive treat.

105. S'mores

Ingredient:

• Graham crackers
• Milk chocolate bars, broken into squares
• Marshmallows

Instructions:

1. Gather all the ingredients and any necessary tools, like skewers or roasting sticks.

2. For each s'more, place a square of chocolate on a graham cracker.

3. Carefully roast a marshmallow over an open flame, such as a campfire or gas stove burner. Keep a close eye on the marshmallow to prevent it from burning.

4. Once the marshmallow is toasted to your desired doneness, quickly place it on top of the chocolate.

5. Top with another graham cracker to make a sandwich.

6. Gently press down to allow the chocolate and marshmallow to melt together.

7. Enjoy the warm, gooey s'more!

Tips for Young Chefs:
• Supervise closely when roasting the marshmallows, as the open flame can be dangerous.
• Demonstrate how to carefully rotate the marshmallow to get an even toasting.
• Have the kids take turns roasting their own marshmallows.
• Encourage creativity by trying different chocolate flavors or adding toppings like crushed graham crackers.
• Discuss food safety, like not eating anything that has fallen on the ground.

S'mores are a classic, easy•to•make treat that young chefs will love. The hands•on assembly and fun of roasting the marshmallows make it a great activity for kids.

106. Chocolate Truffles

Ingredient:

• 8 oz semisweet chocolate, finely chopped
• 1/2 cup heavy cream
• 2 tbsp unsalted butter, softened
• 1/4 tsp vanilla extract
• Cocoa powder, for coating

Instructions:

1. Place the chopped chocolate in a medium heatproof bowl.

2. In a small saucepan, heat the heavy cream over medium heat until it just begins to simmer. Remove from heat.

3. Pour the hot cream over the chopped chocolate and let sit for 2•3 minutes to allow the chocolate to melt.

4. Whisk the mixture gently until smooth and creamy. Stir in the softened butter and vanilla until fully incorporated.

5. Cover the bowl and refrigerate the chocolate ganache for at least 2 hours, until firm.

6. Using a small cookie scoop or spoon, scoop out small portions of the ganache and roll them into 1•inch balls between your palms.

7. Place the truffles on a parchment•lined baking sheet and refrigerate for 30 minutes.

8. Pour some cocoa powder into a shallow bowl. Roll the chilled truffles in the cocoa powder to coat.

9. Store the finished truffles in an airtight container in the refrigerator for up to 1 week.

These homemade chocolate truffles are a delicious and impressive treat that young chefs will enjoy making. The simple ingredients and hands•on preparation make it a fun baking project.

107. Lava Cake

Ingredient:

- 4 oz semisweet chocolate, chopped
- 1/2 cup unsalted butter, plus more for greasing
- 2 large eggs
- 2 large egg yolks
- 1/4 cup granulated sugar
- 2 tbsp all•purpose flour

Instructions:

1. Preheat the oven to 450°F. Grease four 6•oz ramekins with butter and dust with cocoa powder.

2. In a medium heatproof bowl, melt the chopped chocolate and 1/2 cup of butter together over a pot of simmering water, stirring occasionally until smooth. Remove from heat and let cool slightly.

3. In a medium bowl, whisk together the eggs, egg yolks, and sugar until light and fluffy, about 2•3 minutes.

4. Gently fold the melted chocolate mixture and flour into the egg mixture until just combined.

5. Divide the batter evenly among the prepared ramekins.

6. Bake for 8•10 minutes, until the edges are set but the centers are still soft and molten.

7. Carefully invert the cakes onto plates and serve immediately, garnished with powdered sugar, whipped cream, or ice cream if desired.

Tips for Young Chefs:
- Have an adult help with the double boiler setup for melting the chocolate.
- Let the kids measure and whisk the egg and sugar mixture.
- Demonstrate how to gently fold in the chocolate and flour.
- Supervise when filling and baking the ramekins.
- Encourage creativity with different garnishes or sauces.

These decadent molten lava cakes are a fun and impressive dessert that young chefs will enjoy making. The simple steps and hands•on preparation make it a great baking project.

108. Peanut Butter Cookies

Ingredient:

- 1 cup creamy peanut butter
- 1 cup granulated sugar
- 1 large egg
- 1 tsp vanilla extract
- 1/4 tsp salt

Instructions:

1. Preheat the oven to 350°F. Line a baking sheet with parchment paper.

2. In a medium bowl, stir together the peanut butter, sugar, egg, vanilla, and salt until well combined.

3. Scoop rounded tablespoons of dough and place them about 2 inches apart on the prepared baking sheet.

4. Use a fork to gently press a criss•cross pattern into the top of each cookie.

5. Bake for 8•10 minutes, until the cookies are lightly golden around the edges.

6. Allow the cookies to cool on the baking sheet for 5 minutes before transferring to a wire rack to cool completely.

Tips for Young Chefs:
- Let the kids help measure and mix the ingredients.
- Have them scoop the dough onto the baking sheet.
- Demonstrate how to use a fork to make the criss•cross pattern.
- Supervise when putting the cookies in and taking them out of the oven.
- Encourage them to get creative with decorations like sprinkles or chocolate chips.

These classic peanut butter cookies are a simple and delicious recipe that young chefs will enjoy making. The short ingredient list and easy steps make it a great baking project for kids.

109. Mango Sticky Rice

Ingredient:

• 1 cup (200g) short•grain sticky rice (also called sweet rice or glutinous rice)
• 1 cup (240ml) coconut milk
• 1/2 cup (100g) white sugar
• 1/4 tsp salt
• 1•2 ripe mangoes, peeled and sliced
• Toasted sesame seeds for garnish (optional)

For the Coconut Sauce:
• 1/2 cup (120ml) coconut milk
• 2 tbsp white sugar
• 1/4 tsp salt

Instructions:

1. Rinse the sticky rice in a fine mesh strainer until the water runs clear. Soak the rice in water for at least 30 minutes, then drain.

2. In a medium saucepan, combine the 1 cup of coconut milk, 1/2 cup sugar, and 1/4 tsp salt. Bring to a simmer over medium heat, stirring to dissolve the sugar.

3. Add the drained sticky rice and stir. Reduce heat to low, cover and cook for 20•25 minutes, stirring occasionally, until the rice is tender and has absorbed most of the liquid.

4. Remove from heat and let sit, covered, for 10 more minutes. Fluff with a fork.

5. For the coconut sauce, combine the 1/2 cup coconut milk, 2 tbsp sugar, and 1/4 tsp salt in a small saucepan. Heat and stir until the sugar has dissolved. Set aside.

6. To serve, scoop the warm sticky rice into bowls. Top with sliced fresh mango. Drizzle the coconut sauce over the top and sprinkle with toasted sesame seeds if desired.

Enjoy this sweet, creamy, and tropical Thai dessert! The combination of the sticky rice, sweet mango, and rich coconut sauce is simply divine.

110. Pavlova

Ingredient:

- 4 egg whites, at room temperature
- 1 cup (200g) white granulated sugar
- 1 tsp white vinegar
- 1 tsp cornflour (cornstarch)
- 1 tsp vanilla extract
- 300ml heavy cream, whipped
- Fresh fruit for topping (such as berries, kiwi, passionfruit)

Instructions:

1. Preheat the oven to 300ºF (150ºC). Line a baking sheet with parchment paper.

2. In a large clean bowl, beat the egg whites with an electric mixer on high speed until they form soft peaks. Gradually add the sugar, 1•2 tablespoons at a time, beating well after each addition until the meringue is stiff and glossy.

3. Gently fold in the vinegar, cornflour, and vanilla extract until just combined.

4. Spoon the meringue onto the prepared baking sheet, shaping it into a round, flat•topped disk about 8 inches wide and 1•2 inches high.

5. Bake for 60•75 minutes, until the outside is crisp and lightly golden. Turn off the oven and leave the meringue inside with the door closed for an additional hour to cool completely.

6. Once cooled, carefully transfer the meringue to a serving plate. Top with the whipped cream and arrange the fresh fruit on top.

7. Serve immediately or refrigerate until ready to serve. Enjoy!

The key to a successful pavlova is getting the meringue just right • crisp on the outside and soft and marshmallowy on the inside. Experiment with different fruit toppings to find your favorite combination.

111. Pumpkin Roll

Ingredient:

- 3 large eggs
- 1 cup (200g) granulated sugar
- 2/3 cup (160g) canned pumpkin puree
- 3/4 cup (94g) all•purpose flour
- 1 tsp baking powder
- 2 tsp ground cinnamon
- 1/2 tsp ground ginger
- 1/4 tsp ground nutmeg
- 1/4 tsp salt

Filling Ingredients:

- 8 oz (225g) cream cheese, softened
- 1 cup (120g) powdered sugar
- 6 tbsp (85g) unsalted butter, softened
- 1 tsp vanilla extract
- 1/4 tsp salt

Instructions:

1. Preheat oven to 375°F (190°C). Grease a 15x10 inch jelly roll pan and line with parchment paper.

2. In a large bowl, beat the eggs for 5 minutes until thick and lemon•colored. Gradually add the granulated sugar and beat until well combined.

3. Fold in the pumpkin puree until just combined.

4. In a separate bowl, whisk together the flour, baking powder, cinnamon, ginger, nutmeg, and salt.

5. Fold the dry ingredients into the wet ingredients until no dry pockets remain.

6. Spread the batter evenly into the prepared pan. Bake for 13•15 minutes, until the top springs back when lightly touched.

7. Immediately invert the cake onto a clean kitchen towel dusted with powdered sugar. Carefully peel off the parchment paper.

8. Starting from the short end, tightly roll up the cake in the towel. Allow to cool completely, seam•side down.

9. For the filling, beat the cream cheese, powdered sugar, butter, vanilla, and salt until smooth and creamy.

10. Carefully unroll the cooled cake. Spread the cream cheese filling evenly over the surface.

11. Reroll the cake without the towel. Wrap in plastic wrap and refrigerate for at least 1 hour before slicing and serving.

112. Molten Chocolate Cake

Ingredient:

• 6 oz (170g) bittersweet chocolate, chopped
• 1/2 cup (115g) unsalted butter, plus more for greasing
• 3 large eggs
• 3 large egg yolks
• 1/3 cup (67g) granulated sugar
• 2 tbsp all•purpose flour
• Pinch of salt
• Powdered sugar for dusting (optional)
• Vanilla ice cream or whipped cream for serving (optional)

Instructions:

1. Preheat the oven to 450ºF (230ºC). Grease four 6•oz ramekins or custard cups with butter and dust with cocoa powder.

2. In a medium heatproof bowl set over a saucepan of simmering water, melt the chocolate and 1/2 cup butter, stirring occasionally, until smooth. Remove from heat and let cool slightly.

3. In a medium bowl, whisk together the eggs, egg yolks, and granulated sugar until light and fluffy, about 2•3 minutes.

4. Fold the melted chocolate mixture into the egg mixture until just combined. Then fold in the flour and salt until no dry pockets remain.

5. Divide the batter evenly among the prepared ramekins. Bake for 8•10 minutes, until the edges are set but the centers are still soft and molten.

6. Carefully run a knife around the edges of the cakes and invert them onto plates. Dust with powdered sugar if desired.

7. Serve the molten chocolate cakes immediately, with a scoop of vanilla ice cream or whipped cream on the side.

The key is to not overbake the cakes so the centers stay warm and gooey. Enjoy this rich, decadent chocolate dessert!

113. Cinnamon Rolls

Ingredient:

- 1 cup (240ml) warm milk (110°F/45°C)
- 2 1/4 tsp (7g) active dry yeast
- 1/2 cup (100g) granulated sugar
- 1/4 cup (57g) unsalted butter, softened
- 1 tsp salt
- 1 egg
- 4 1/2 cups (563g) all•purpose flour, plus more for dusting

Filling Ingredients:

- 1 cup (200g) brown sugar, packed
- 2 tbsp ground cinnamon
- 1/3 cup (75g) unsalted butter, softened

Cream Cheese Frosting:

- 4 oz (115g) cream cheese, softened
- 1/4 cup (57g) unsalted butter, softened
- 1 1/2 cups (180g) powdered sugar
- 1/2 tsp vanilla extract
- 1/8 tsp salt

Instructions:

1. In a large bowl, combine the warm milk, yeast, and 1 tbsp of the sugar. Let sit for 5•10 minutes until foamy.

2. Add the remaining sugar, butter, salt, egg, and 2 cups of the flour. Mix until a shaggy dough forms.

3. Turn dough out onto a lightly floured surface and knead for 5•7 minutes, adding more flour as needed, until smooth and elastic.

4. Place dough in a lightly greased bowl, cover, and let rise for 1•2 hours, until doubled in size.

5. Punch down the dough to release air bubbles. On a lightly floured surface, roll the dough into a 16x21 inch rectangle.

6. Spread the 1/3 cup softened butter over the dough. In a small bowl, mix the brown sugar and cinnamon. Sprinkle evenly over the butter.

7. Tightly roll up the dough, starting from the long side. Cut into 12 equal pieces.

8. Place rolls in a greased 9x13 inch baking pan. Cover and let rise for 30 minutes.

9. Preheat oven to 350°F (177°C). Bake for 20•25 minutes until golden brown.

10. Make the frosting: Beat the cream cheese and butter until smooth. Add powdered sugar, vanilla, and salt and beat until fluffy. Spread the warm cinnamon rolls with the cream cheese frosting. Serve warm.

114. Baklava

Ingredient:

Filling:
• 2 cups (240g) chopped walnuts or pistachios
• 1 cup (200g) granulated sugar
• 1 tsp ground cinnamon

Phyllo Dough:
• 16 sheets phyllo dough, thawed if frozen
• 1 cup (230g) unsalted butter, melted

Syrup:
• 1 cup (240ml) honey
• 1 cup (200g) granulated sugar
• 1 cup (240ml) water
• 1 tbsp lemon juice

Instructions:

1. Preheat oven to 350°F (177°C). Grease a 9x13 inch baking dish.

2. Make the filling: In a medium bowl, mix together the chopped nuts, 1 cup sugar, and cinnamon. Set aside.

3. Lay 1 sheet of phyllo dough in the prepared baking dish and brush with melted butter. Repeat with 7 more sheets, brushing each with butter.

4. Spread half of the nut filling evenly over the phyllo layers.

5. Top with 8 more sheets of phyllo, brushing each with butter.

6. Spread the remaining nut filling over the phyllo. Top with the final 8 sheets of phyllo, brushing each with butter.

7. Using a sharp knife, cut the unbaked baklava into squares or diamonds. Bake for 35•45 minutes, until the phyllo is golden brown.

8. While the baklava bakes, make the syrup: In a small saucepan, combine the honey, 1 cup sugar, water, and lemon juice. Bring to a boil, then reduce heat and simmer for 10 minutes.

9. Remove the baked baklava from the oven and immediately pour the hot syrup over the top. Allow to cool completely, at least 4 hours or overnight.

10.. Once cooled, cut along the pre•cut lines to serve. Enjoy the sweet, nutty, and flaky baklava!

The key is to use plenty of butter between the phyllo layers and to pour the hot syrup over the just•baked baklava so it soaks in. This makes for an incredibly rich and delicious Greek dessert.

115. Almond Biscotti

Ingredient:

• 2 cups (250g) all•purpose flour
• 1 1/2 tsp baking powder
• 1/4 tsp salt
• 3/4 cup (150g) granulated sugar
• 1/2 cup (115g) unsalted butter, softened
• 2 large eggs
• 1 tsp vanilla extract
• 1 cup (150g) whole almonds, toasted and chopped

Instructions:

1. Preheat the oven to 350°F (177°C). Line a large baking sheet with parchment paper.

2. In a medium bowl, whisk together the flour, baking powder, and salt. Set aside.

3. In a large bowl, beat the sugar and butter together until light and fluffy, about 2•3 minutes. Beat in the eggs one at a time, then stir in the vanilla.

4. Gradually mix the dry ingredients into the wet ingredients until just combined. Fold in the chopped toasted almonds.

5. Divide the dough in half. On a lightly floured surface, shape each half into a 12•inch long log, about 1•inch thick.

6. Transfer the logs to the prepared baking sheet, spacing them a few inches apart.

7. Bake for 25 minutes, until the logs are lightly golden brown. Remove from the oven and let cool for 5 minutes.

8. Using a sharp knife, slice each log diagonally into 1/2•inch thick slices. Arrange the slices cut•side down on the baking sheet.

9. Bake for an additional 10•12 minutes, flipping the biscotti halfway, until golden brown and crisp. Remove from the oven and let cool completely on the baking sheet before serving.

The biscotti will continue to crisp up as they cool. Store in an airtight container for up to 2 weeks.

*Congratulations on reaching the end of **The Complete Cookbook for Young Chefs!**
By now, you've conquered an array of delicious and nutritious meals, from
breakfast to dinner, and everything in between. You've explored new flavors, honed
your cooking skills, and hopefully discovered a newfound passion for creating
amazing dishes in your kitchen.*

*This cookbook was designed to be more than just a collection of recipes. It's a
resource to inspire confidence, creativity, and a love for cooking that will serve you
well throughout your life. You've learned essential techniques, picked up handy tips,
and mastered recipes that you can proudly share with family and friends.*

*Remember, cooking is an ongoing journey of exploration and learning. Don't be
afraid to experiment with new ingredients, modify recipes to suit your taste, and
continue building on the skills you've developed. The kitchen is your playground,
and every meal is an opportunity to create something wonderful.*

*Thank you for allowing this book to be part of your culinary adventure. We hope it
has brought you joy, delicious meals, and a sense of accomplishment. Keep
cooking, keep experimenting, and most importantly, keep having fun in the kitchen.*

Happy cooking, and bon appétit!

9 798329 663907